I0605286

"*Seeking Sanctuary, Finding Shalom* offers readers a well-researched and beautifully written synthesis of theological insight and cutting-edge theory in psychology. Swinton's work provides a vision for mental health based upon a biblical understanding of shalom, as it is manifest in peace with oneself, with others, with creation, and with God. Swinton also raises significant overarching issues about mental health in the context of the broader culture, asking the necessary question, 'Could Western culture be bad for our mental health?' He highlights the role of social injustice in the rates of mental health impairment as well as market influences on the business of mental health treatment. His work is theory-rich and grounded in eschatological hope, at the same time that it offers practical responses to the challenge of understanding mental health in a Western world context."

—MARCIA WEBB, *Associate Professor of Psychology, Seattle Pacific University*

"John Swinton invites us to reimagine mental health through a theological vision of shalom, peace, and yet much more than 'just' peace. Mental health, according to this vision, is inherently relational and theological, being concerned with peace within and between minds, peace with creation, and peace with God. *Seeking Sanctuary, Finding Shalom* offers a siren call for decommodification, kindness, and compassion in mental healthcare."

—CHRISTOPHER C. H. COOK, *Emeritus Professor, Institute for Medical Humanities, Durham University*

"When Pope John XXIII began the Second Vatican Council, he is said to have thrown open a window in order to 'let the fresh air of the Spirit blow through.' I think that John Swinton must have opened his window when he was writing this book. With characteristic insight, Swinton connects the dots between the personal, interpersonal, political, economic, and ecological causes of mental illness. In so doing, he shows how moving from an understanding of mental health as the absence of mental illness to the idea of mental health as shalom overcomes alienating dichotomies, allowing us to see more clearly the systemic causes of mental illness and help us to overcome them."

—TASIA SCRUTTON, *Associate Professor in Philosophy and Religion, University of Leeds*

"In a time when mental health concerns and therapeutic pursuits are everywhere—like our social media feeds—we need a faithful and wise guide. There is no one more fit to lead us than John Swinton. With his usual depth, creativity, and pastoral sensitivity, *Seeking Sanctuary, Finding Shalom* adds to Swinton's important corpus. The pastoral and theological insights of this book will form and direct you."

—ANDREW ROOT, *Professor and Carrie Olson Baalson Chair of Youth and Family Ministry, Luther Seminary*

SEEKING SANCTUARY, FINDING SHALOM

Toward a Deeper Practical Theology of Mental Health

JOHN SWINTON
ANGELA H. REED, EDITOR

BAYLOR UNIVERSITY PRESS

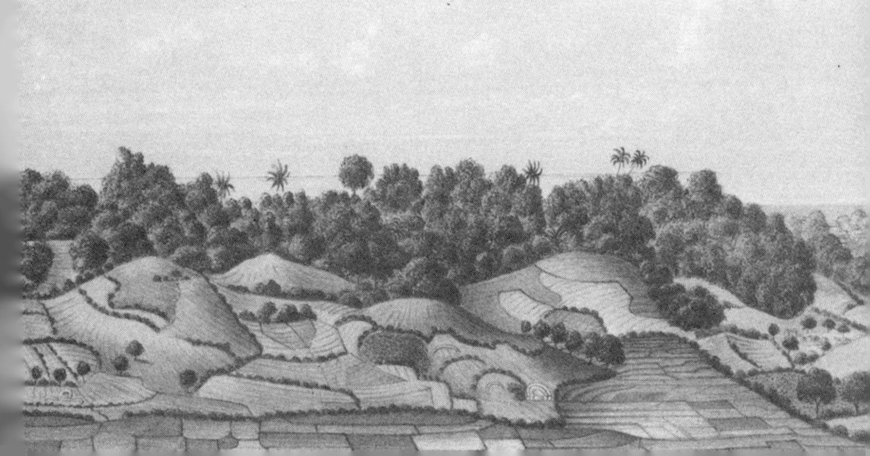

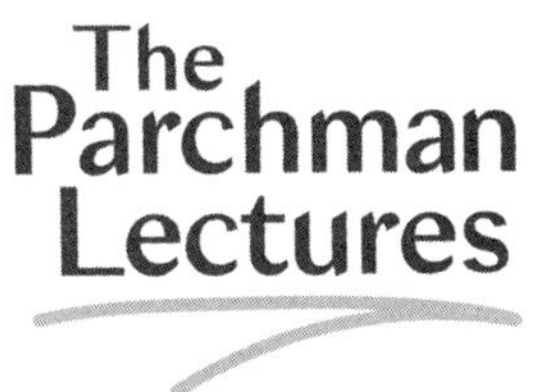

The Truett Parchman Lectures

Kimlyn J. Bender
Series Editor

The Truett Parchman Lecture series, a joint venture in publishing between George W. Truett Theological Seminary and Baylor University Press, seeks to make the Parchman Endowed Lectures available to a wide audience. The Parchman Lectures are given annually at the Seminary and are made possible by an endowment gifted by Leo and Gloriana Parchman. These lectures bring world-renowned theologians to the Baylor University campus and enable Truett Theological Seminary to make a significant contribution to the realm of theological scholarship and dialogue as well as to the life of the church.

The Parchman Lectures were inaugurated in 1999 with those given by Jürgen Moltmann. In the ensuing years, the lectures have been given by scholars such as Richard Bauckham, Walter Brueggemann, James Forbes, Justo González, Bill Leonard, Alister McGrath, Margaret Mitchell, Richard Mouw, Eugene Peterson, John Polkinghorne, Dana Robert, Fleming Rutledge, Lamin Sanneh, James K. A. Smith, Geoffrey Wainwright, and N. T. Wright.

Also Available in the Series

By the Word Worked
Fleming Rutledge

Series and cover design by Elyxandra Encarnación
Cover art: North coast near Semarang by Franz Wilhelm Junghuhn, 1854. Public domain.

The Library of Congress has cataloged this book under ISBN 978-1-4813-2471-7.
Library of Congress Control Number: 2025939701

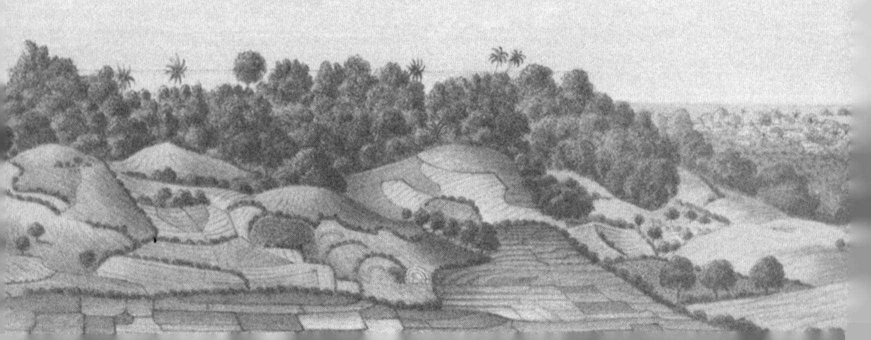

CONTENTS

Foreword xi
Angela H. Reed

Acknowledgments xix

Introduction 1

1 What Is Mental Health? 5
Shalom as a Guiding Vision

2 Peace Within Minds Requires Peace Between Minds 27
Why the Inner Life Is Always Already Relational

3 Finding Peace with Creation 67
Culture, Systems, Politics, and the Land

4 Finding Peace with God 109

A Deeper, Kinder Theology of Mental Health

Postscript 147

Being Where Our Feet Are

FOREWORD
ANGELA H. REED

Researchers estimate that at least one in five adults in the United States lives with a mental illness. The prevalence of mental health problems among young adults is even higher.[1] These statistics are certainly not unique to American studies. The numbers are staggering, and they leave us with critical questions. What do we mean by "mental illness" and "mental health?" Who and what determines if a mind is healthy in the context of our mental healthcare systems? What does the Christian tradition teach us

[1] See https://www.nimh.nih.gov/health/statistics/mental-illness. The data suggest that more than one in three young adults lives with a mental illness. Significant numbers of children and youth are impacted by mental illness as well. See https://www.cdc.gov/children-mental-health/data-research/index.html.

about a healthy mind? How might God be calling us to nurture healthy minds together in connection with God and all creation? These queries are just the beginning of a much-needed practical and theological conversation about mental health rooted in the life and ministry of the church. Ultimately, congregations and their leaders want to participate in mental healthcare in some way. Many ministers and lay people are eager to support individuals and their families facing mental illnesses, but they may not be equipped theologically or practically to meet these pressing needs.

I can think of no better place to raise these questions than a theological school filled with ministers-in-training taught by a scholar with the wisdom and experience of Dr. John Swinton. We were thrilled to welcome Dr. Swinton to George W. Truett Theological Seminary and Baylor University to offer the Parchman Lectures on the topic of mental health and practical theology. Dr. Swinton himself embodies a deeper, kinder way of being as he interacts with people and as he writes. He begins by offering us a definition of mental health rooted in *shalom* that is wholly relational, involving connection with God, self, others, and all creation. A deeper, kinder understanding of mental health does not focus primarily on a cure that requires the absence of ill-health. A healthful understanding of *shalom*, especially for those living with mental illness throughout their lives, looks beyond biology alone, resisting a quick fix in order to tend well to the whole person.

Dr. Swinton goes on to challenge traditional Western understandings of the mind that are inherently individualistic by discussing interpersonal neurobiology, anthropology, and extended mind theory. This interdisciplinary dialogue is relatively new in practical theology and mental health studies. It challenges reliance on market-based medical models of care and current diagnostic criteria as the sole approaches to addressing the health and well-being of the whole person. These insights align beautifully with the biblical witness, particularly the Pauline vision of the body of Christ. The people of God are invited to take up a remarkable call of accountability for the health of one another's minds. The wisdom inherent in *shalom* and the gifts of the body of Christ give us normative frameworks for redefining mental health, for responding to loneliness with kind-ness, even kinship, and for creating peace-filled sanctuaries in the midst of suffering. Perhaps one of the most forward-thinking challenges involves expanding our vision beyond the individual and even corporate mind of today to the ecological crisis and the well-being of minds tomorrow and beyond. These chapters certainly challenge us to think more deeply about the nature of mental health and hear afresh the Christian call to Christ-like caring.

The concerns Dr. Swinton wisely raises about individualized understandings of the mind and healthcare systems are part of a larger trajectory of declining social connections and social networks over decades in the Western world. In recent years, the former Surgeon General of the United States, Dr. Vivek Murthy, has issued alerts regarding a loneliness epidemic impacting about half of adults. The physical, mental, and emotional impacts are acute. The physical health data alone suggest that mortality rates are akin to smoking up to fifteen cigarettes a day. Active participation in positive relationship-building through religious organizations, civic groups, friendship circles, and other emotional support systems has declined significantly. It is not surprising that people are overwhelmed by a sense of carrying the daily burdens of life alone.[2] These factors make it even more difficult to nurture healthy

[2] *Our Epidemic of Loneliness and Isolation: The U.S. Surgeon General's Advisory on the Healing Effects of Social Connection and Community* (U.S. Public Health Service, 2023). See also Vivek Murthy, *Together: The Healing Power of Human Connection in a Sometimes Lonely World* (HarperCollins, 2020).

minds together. Dr. Swinton's practical theological vision for healthcare rooted in spiritual community could not come at a better time.

This insightful work also invites us to reflect upon stories of mental healthcare arising in our own social, cultural, and spiritual contexts. I have been pondering the journeys of two women in the small farming community I grew up in. Both struggled with significant mental illness and had frequent stays in the local psychiatric facility (a faith-based healthcare organization begun by a community of churches). As a child, I remember thinking that they seemed different somehow, and I did not know what to say or do around them. Yet I noticed that my mother treated them just as she did her other friends, and I tried to do the same. I came to understand that she saw beyond the illnesses to the people they were with hopes and dreams, children and families, like many others in our community. These women were her friends, not projects to fix or problems to solve. One lived down the road from us and had significant needs beyond friendship. Over the years, she received food from the farm, snow clearing, lawn mowing, home and car repairs, and other quiet means of support. These matters were rarely discussed, and the responsibility was passed down to the next generation. At times, my mother's friend was not easy to be with, but she was "kin" and one of the strongest women of faith and prayer I have ever met. When I think of Dr. Swinton's vision for well-being in community despite a lifetime of mental illness, I think of these women.

It is my hope and prayer that the pastoral wisdom filling this volume will challenge all of us to reframe and expand our understanding of mental health for the purposes of genuine healing that creates deepening connection with God, others, self, and all creation. As we consider the persons we know and love, those we work with, live next to, or worship alongside, may we discern how best to become true communities of sanctuary, *ekklesia* small and large, that contribute to the well-being of minds and of all creation now and into the future.

ACKNOWLEDGMENTS

Writing this book has been a journey deeply rooted in relationships, collaboration, and a shared vision. I am deeply thankful to my family and friends for their steadfast support and encouragement throughout this process.

To my wife, Alison, your unwavering love and understanding have been a constant source of strength and inspiration. Thank you for your patience and for always being a sanctuary of peace and joy in my life. To my children, your laughter, kindness, and grounding presence always remind me of the importance of balance and perspective in all things. I am also deeply indebted to Daniel Whitehead, the CEO of Sanctuary Mental Health Ministries, whose friendship, insights, and commitment to reshaping mental healthcare within the Christian community have influenced me over the years we have known each other. To my editors, Kimlyn Bender and Angela Reed, your expertise, wisdom, and dedication have been invaluable. Thank you for believing in this work and helping to bring it to fruition. To my friends, whose kindness and encouragement have buoyed me along the way, thank you for walking this journey with me. Your presence has enriched this work in ways words cannot fully express. The book began as the Parchman lectures I delivered at Baylor University in 2023. I am grateful to the faculty for the invitation that allowed me to develop new ideas and expand my thinking around mental health.

The heart of this book was formed through these relationships, a testament to the power of community, collaboration, and shared hope.

One thing readers of this book may not know is that I am a musician and a songwriter. My album, *Beautiful Songs About Difficult Things*, is a helpful accompaniment to some of the themes and issues that emerge from this book. You can find it on whatever streaming service you use. I hope it is helpful.

INTRODUCTION

Imagine a world where the very systems and beliefs designed to protect and promote mental health are, in reality, causing harm—perpetuating ideologies and practices that deepen the wounds they claim to heal. In this world, cultural assumptions that seem neutral instead shape and fuel a mental health crisis that transcends individuals, embedding suffering deep within the fabric of society. Efforts to promote mental health in such a world unintentionally sustain oppressive systems that generate ill health. Resilience, often celebrated as a virtue, becomes a tool not for liberation but for survival—equipping individuals to endure harmful structures rather than challenging or transforming them. In this world, mental health experiences vary drastically across cultures, with Western societies seemingly facing the most significant struggles with conditions such as depression and schizophrenia. And this world bears witness to escalating ecological crises through phones, tablets, and screens; people seem not to notice the profound mental and emotional toll of such devastation on our collective well-being. This book argues that this world is not hypothetical—it is *our* world. It invites us to confront these unsettling realities and consider bold, sometimes unusual questions about mental health, what it is, what disrupts it, and how Christians might act faithfully in response.

At heart, this book invites readers to think theologically about mental health, not merely as an individual concern but as a matter intricately connected to the collective body of humanity and the welfare of creation. In what follows, I suggest that to understand the nature of faithful Christian mental healthcare, we need to examine not only what occurs within individual minds—important as that is—but also what transpires *between* minds and throughout all of creation. The ways we structure creation—relational, social, cultural, political, spiritual—profoundly impact our mental health. Failing to acknowledge the broader, more holistic dimensions of mental healthcare risks engaging in dangerous palliation—easing the severity of pain or disease without addressing the root cause—rather than fostering genuine healing that cultivates a peaceable connection with God, self, others, and creation. Faithful mental healthcare requires us to look inward, outward, and upward simultaneously. While this is a more complex task, it yields life-giving rewards.

1
WHAT IS MENTAL HEALTH?

Shalom as a Guiding Vision

Mental health is a complex, contextual, and contested notion. While it can be helpful, it can also paradoxically be detrimental to our well-being. Therefore, I will begin by outlining in detail the understanding of mental health that underpins this book, that of *shalom*. Shalom means peace, but as we will see, it is a form of peace that is crucial for our understanding of mental health and mental healthcare.

DOES MENTAL HEALTH REFER TO THE ABSENCE OR THE PRESENCE OF SOMETHING?

It is tempting to define mental health by what it is not, such as: *Mental health is not mental ill-health.* We might, for example, say that mental health is present when symptoms are absent. When I am not anxious, depressed, hearing voices, and so forth, I am mentally well. When these symptoms are present,

I am mentally unwell. Here, mental health becomes a goal achieved by alleviating symptoms and cultivating a certain kind of peace (often defined by the absence of stress or anxiety and the presence of happiness and emotional stability). Such an oppositional definition assumes that mental health and mental ill-health cannot coexist in the same space.[1]

This type of binary thinking influences our expectations regarding appropriate intervention and the nature of healing. It also drives us toward a singular goal and desire: *to discover paths from ill health to health*. This, in turn, raises specific expectations of medicine and psychiatry (and indeed the healing ministry of the church). We assume that psychiatry or psychology are the disciplines we turn to when we want our problems solved, fixed, and mended. When

[1] A mediating position is the idea of a mental health continuum. Here the assumption is that everyone is on a continuum moving from mental health at one end to mental ill-health at the other. This helps break down assumptions that people with mental health challenges are radically different from those who do not have such challenges. This is a helpful position, but unless one is clear about what mental health and ill-health are, it is not clear what one is moving between. Corey L. M. Keyes, "The Mental Health Continuum: From Languishing to Flourishing in Life," *Journal of Health and Social Behavior* 43, no. 2 (2002): 207–22.

something goes wrong with us and our mental health is disrupted, we look to these disciplines to help us return to a healthier state, usually defined by the presence or absence of symptoms and certain negative emotions. Mental health is defined in terms of *the lack of illness or suffering.* We *expect* the mental healthcare disciplines to fix us because we assume that the "health" in mental healthcare pertains to a movement away from ill health. All of this seems quite natural, normal, and, in many ways, desirable. The power of medicine and the healing balm of psychiatry lies in their ability *to* bring about relief from suffering. Helping people move away from pain and suffering is commendable and laudable, as long as that is a possibility. This is undoubtedly a good thing. However, sadly, for many living with enduring mental health challenges, the idea of being fixed and mended is a desirable but unattainable goal. Some people will have to live with their mental health challenges for their entire lives.

When you can't move away from your troubles

The problem is that if health is defined by the absence of, or movement away from, illness, many people will be destined to live their lives labeled as "unhealthy." Those living with enduring forms of physical and mental ill-health find themselves judged as perpetually ill.[2] Even when they feel well, the assumption persists that they are in remission, always anticipating and waiting for the time when their condition will return.[3] In this perspective,

[2] This observation resonates with the sociologist Talcott Parson's idea of the sick role. Here, the sick person is exempted from normal social roles, is not responsible for their condition, and is obligated to seek competent medical help and cooperate toward getting well. In other words, being ill has social meaning and implications for being in the world that transcend the particularities of any given ailment. Talcott Parsons, *The Social System* (The Free Press, 1951), 428–79.

[3] The idea of always being ill comes from the medical sociologist Arthur Frank. He proposed the idea of a "remission society" to describe the unique experiences of those living with chronic or recurring illnesses. In a remission society, the goal is not necessarily a "cure" or full recovery, but rather an ongoing process of managing symptoms and maintaining a good quality of life. People living in a remission society vacillate between periods of illness and wellness. Their lives are punctuated by remission and relapse. This requires learning to live with uncertainty and appreciating the temporary reprieves from symptoms. Hope is focused on making the most of the "good days." The experience forges new identities and social roles as people cope with their illnesses and share their experiences. It highlights the need for healthcare that treats patients holistically, not just targeting disease. Attention is given to healing and well-being. Arthur W. Frank, *The Wounded Storyteller: Body, Illness, and Ethics* (University of Chicago Press, 1995).

mental health, understood as the absence of ill-health, becomes an unachievable goal for those living with enduring mental health challenges. This, in turn, divides human beings into two categories: those who are well and those who are perpetually unwell; those who need treatment to attain mental health, and those for whom there is no curative treatment. Understood in this way, wellness is at best a temporary state, with chronic unwellness presumed, implicitly or explicitly, to be for some a permanent condition. This perception makes the experience of mental ill-health particularly fear-inducing for "the well." The realm of illness becomes a strange place that looms ominously on the edges of everyone's life, waiting patiently for the moment when we might tumble into its unfamiliar and frightening world, never to return to the land of the well. This, in turn, encourages the stigmatization, alienation, and marginalization of those who must live with mental ill-health throughout their lives.

Deprioritizing care

This way of thinking about health in general and mental health in particular not only puts immense pressure on medicine and psychiatry to view cure as their primary measure of success, but it also steers our cultural and political values and investments. Our healthcare system's emphasis on *curing* diseases and controlling symptoms often comes at the expense of *caring for* and treating whole persons. This manifests in several ways: the prioritization of pharmaceuticals over holistic coping strategies, disproportionate spending on curative treatments rather than ongoing care, insurance coverage favoring quick fixes, and research focusing on biological factors rather than social determinants. This imbalance stems from a narrow vision of health as merely the absence of illness, placing pressure on medical professionals, researchers, and funders to emphasize primarily or even solely symptom control instead of quality of life.

Importantly, this perspective on health biases society towards seeking individual solutions instead of addressing systemic issues. Mental health challenges are framed as occurrences affecting individuals rather than resulting from situations imposed by broader social pressures. Mental health treatments become individualized and commodified, concentrating on alleviating *personal* symptoms. Mental healthcare evolves into a market where significant profits are generated to manage people's problems while neglecting the societal changes needed to prioritize well-being over symptom control. As we will see in chapter 2, when mental healthcare gets ensnared in the realm of commodities and markets, it can negatively impact individuals' mental health.

The central thrust of this book is that we need a new approach to understanding mental health—one that considers the intricate and foundational roots of human psychological suffering, which I will describe as "creational." This approach offers a model of human flourishing that is not limited to the absence of pain, suffering, or distress but is instead defined by the transformative presence of God. Such a model takes human suffering very seriously but understands its roots within a broader creational framework. This approach seeks not only to address the immediacies of pain and suffering but also to view those realities within the context of Jesus's cosmic mission to reconcile himself with *all* things. Participating in that reconciliation and addressing the aspects within creation that contribute to mental distress is a significant marker of faithful Christian mental healthcare. I propose that the roots of such a perspective lie in the biblical concept of shalom.

MENTAL HEALTH AS SHALOM

Elsewhere I have written extensively on the relationship between shalom and mental health.[4] Here I

[4] John Swinton, *From Bedlam to Shalom: Towards a Practical Theology of Human Nature—Interpersonal Relationships and Mental Health Care* (Peter Lang, 2000);

focus on a few key aspects of shalom that can frame and guide the arguments of this book. The concept of health within the biblical narrative is not encapsulated by the modern biomedical perspective, which, as I have suggested, tends to define health by the absence of ill-health. Instead, the Bible offers the term *shalom*. Shalom is a Hebrew word often translated as "peace," but its meaning is much broader than the mere absence of conflict or distress. It signifies a state of completeness, wholeness, and harmony that is part of God's original design for creation (Gen 1). Shalom is the human being dwelling in peace in all his or her relationships: with God, with self, with fellow human beings, and with creation. Shalom, as portrayed in Isaiah 11:6–8, is when

> the wolf shall dwell with the lamb,
> and the leopard shall lie down with the young
> goat,
> and the calf and the young lion and the fatling
> together;
> and a little child shall lead them.
> The cow and the bear shall graze;

---

idem, *Resurrecting the Person: Friendship and the Care of People with Severe Mental Health Problems* (Abingdon, 2000); idem, *Finding Jesus in the Storm: The Spiritual Lives of Christians with Mental Health Challenges* (Eerdmans, 2020).

> their young shall lie down together;
> and the lion shall eat straw like the ox.
> The nursing child shall play over the hole of
> the cobra,
> and the weaned child shall put his hand on
> the adder's den. (NRSV)

Shalom is not an ideal, a social movement, or an ideology. *Shalom is a person*: Jesus. In Ephesians 2:14–17 the Apostle Paul informs us that

> he is our peace in his flesh he has made both into one and has broken down the dividing wall, that is, the hostility between us, abolishing the law with its commandments and ordinances, that he might create in himself one new humanity in place of the two, thus making peace, and might reconcile both to God in one body through the cross, thus putting to death that hostility through it. So he came and proclaimed peace to you who were far off and peace to those who were near. (NRSV)

Here, Paul's use of the Greek term *eirene* parallels the Hebrew *shalom*, depicting Jesus as the embodiment of this peace. *Jesus Christ is our peace.* In him, disparate groups are united, walls of hostility are torn down, and peace is proclaimed to all people.

Jesus brings peace and leaves peace with us. In John 14:27, he states: "Peace I leave with you; my peace I give you. I do not give to you as the world gives. Do not let your hearts be troubled, and do not be afraid" (NIV). Jesus imparts his shalom—that is, himself-in-the-Spirit—to his disciples. As followers of Jesus, we are by definition called to be a people of peace who, in the Spirit of Jesus, strive to take what is broken and restore it to wholeness.

Shalom and God's presence

This view of Jesus as shalom and of peace as the goal of his followers has important implications for the ways in which we might think about mental health. Shalom encompasses more than personal happiness, inner harmony, or mental tranquility. Shalom is deeply connected to the means by which we achieve such things: *the presence of God*. It is as we encounter the presence of God that we experience true health. Health is not and does not require the absence of illness. Rather, it has to do with learning what it means to encounter God's presence even amidst unrelieved suffering.

We find this kind of health illustrated in the Psalter, particularly in the Lament Psalms. Psalm 13, for example, discusses the human longing to find

God amidst suffering and the joy of discovering God even when that suffering remains unexplained and unresolved.

> How long, Lord? Will you forget me forever?
> How long will you hide your face from me?
> How long must I bear pain in my soul
> and have sorrow in my heart all day long?
> How long shall my enemy be exalted over me?
>
> Consider and answer me, O Lord my God!
> Give light to my eyes, or I will sleep the sleep of death,
> and my enemy will say, "I have prevailed";
> my foes will rejoice because I am shaken.
>
> But I trusted in your steadfast love;
> my heart shall rejoice in your salvation.
> I will sing to the Lord,
> because he has dealt bountifully with me.
> (NRSV)

Even those psalms that do not culminate in worship remind us of God's presence in the midst of darkness and disconnection. Psalm 88 ends, "You have taken from me friend and neighbor—darkness is my closest friend" (NIV). The sense of hopelessness and disconnection from God is palpable. And yet, this psalm is a prayer. The psalmist does not speak into the void. He addresses a God with whom he cannot, at that moment, connect.

This way of thinking about health and mental health issues challenges Western cultural norms. Imagine a scenario in which an Olympic medalist stands on the podium holding aloft a gold medal. Culturally, the athlete seems to embody health. Yet, if shalom is our model of health, they might actually be deeply unhealthy if they are separated from God and focused only on things that edify themselves. They *appear* healthy, but they may not be. By the same token, someone could be deeply troubled by hearing voices, seeing things that others cannot see, or bearing the social weight of a stigmatized and alienating diagnosis such as schizophrenia, and yet be very healthy inasmuch as their relationship with God anchors them amid their storms, and their relationships with others keep them bound to the body of Christ even when they are struggling. This final point is important. Shalom is a *communal* concept. *It is something we do together*. There may be times when an individual cannot hold on to God, but if we take the body of Christ seriously, then we believe that others can hold on to them through prayers, presence, and persevering friendships.

Shalom as mental health orients us toward the importance of focusing on a person's relationship with God, not as an added extra but as a primary marker of health. It also means that those whom a biomedical model might name as chronically unwell can, in fact, find health and recovery if recovery is defined in terms of people being helped to achieve their life goals and hold on to God in the midst of difficulties.

Shalom as a place of justice

From the perspective of shalom, true peace is not merely personal harmony but encompasses a dynamic relationship with God, others, and creation, reflecting the interconnectedness of all things in God's good design.[5] While societal and creational harmony enrich shalom, they are not its preconditions. These aspects of shalom remain integral yet elusive in a broken world. Inner peace cannot depend on achieving perfect harmony, which lies beyond human capacity. Instead, it is grounded in the sustaining presence of God, who remains with us even amidst injustice and disharmony. Shalom can

[5] The thing that connects is Jesus: "For God was pleased to have all his fullness dwell in him, and through him to reconcile to himself all things, whether things on earth or things in heaven, by making peace through his blood, shed on the cross" (Col 1:19–20 NIV).

be experienced in the midst of brokenness because it is ultimately rooted in a reconciled relationship with God.[6] It manifests when we are at peace within ourselves, when we seek harmony with others, and when we live in faithful alignment with creation—each an expression of God's overarching shalom.[7]

Justice is central to shalom. Nicholas Wolterstorff notes that shalom is impaired when a "society is a collection of individuals all out to make their own way in the world. And of course there can . . . be delight in community only when justice reigns, only when human beings no longer oppress one another."[8] *There can be no shalom without justice, no mental health without fairness.* Wolterstorff continues:

> Shalom cannot be secured in an unjust situation by managing to get all concerned to feel content with their lot in life. Even if poor people were

[6] "I have told you these things, so that in me you may have peace. In this world you will have trouble. But take heart! I have overcome the world" (John 16:33 NIV).

[7] This theme of "shalom as harmony" is developed more fully from an Indigenous perspective in Randy Woodley, *Shalom and the Community of Creation: An Indigenous Vision* (Eerdmans, 2012).

[8] Nicholas Wolterstorff, Clarence W. Joldersma, and Gloria Goris Stronks, *Educating for Shalom: Essays on Christian Higher Education* (Eerdmans, 2004), 70.

> happy to be poor, shalom would not be present. Even if the racially abused, the gender oppressed, the excluded, the migrant, the stranger were happy with their position in life, shalom would not be present.[9]

This is an important point. One of the insights we have gained from liberation theologians is that oppression is not always immediately recognized by those who experience it. Often, people who have been oppressed need to have their consciousness raised so that they can perceive the injustice of their situation. When they realize the true nature of their plight, they are empowered to rise up and begin addressing it. The dynamics of power in the world make issues of freedom and choice complex and often opaque. Justice, however, is not determined by whether someone recognizes or complains about injustice—it is determined by what is righteous in the eyes of God. A fundamental aspect of faithful mental healthcare, and a key task of this book, is to help raise awareness of the often-hidden intersections between mental health and injustice. These connections may not be obvious until they are brought into focus. When injustice is unveiled, it can

[9] Wolterstorff, Joldersma, and Stronks, *Educating for Shalom*, 71.

be confronted. Shalom, then, is not a placid, insipid, idealistic dream. Nor is it a call to rise above suffering and injustice. Rather, it is a call to confront and resist it. This process of conscientization and resistance is an essential dynamic of this book.

Mental health and the cosmic Christ

There is a crucial cosmic dimension to the work of Jesus and his shalomic movement within creation that is vital for mental health. In Colossians 1:19–20 Paul informs us that "God was pleased to have all his fullness dwell in him, and through him to reconcile to himself all things, whether things on earth or things in heaven, by making peace through his blood, shed on the cross" (NIV). Jesus's mission of peace aims to reconcile *all* things to himself. His reconciling work seeks to redeem all of creation. This involves bringing together aspects of creation that have been fragmented and damaged, restoring them to their proper harmony. When one aspect of creation falters, it affects all other aspects—dissonance and damage within creation lead to dissonance and damage within individuals and communities. As a result, mental health is inevitably influenced by the condition of creation. Therefore, engaging with the cosmic, reconciliatory dimensions of Jesus's mission is profoundly significant for mental healthcare. I will return to this in more detail in chapter 3.

Mental health and shalom

In light of these initial reflections on mental health and shalom, we can consider Christian mental healthcare as comprising four interconnecting aspects:

(1) *Peace Within Minds:* This dimension emphasizes the needs of individuals and explores how to foster a sense of internal harmony that enables people to live well, even amid psychological distress. Historically, this has been the primary focus of mental healthcare within the church.

(2) *Peace Between Minds:* Internal harmony cannot be fully understood apart from the interconnectedness of human bodies and, importantly, as we will see, human minds. The dynamics *between* minds—our relationships, interactions, and shared experiences—play a crucial role in shaping what happens *within* individual minds. Peace between minds involves fostering relationships of mutual respect, understanding, and care, recognizing that the quality of our connections with others profoundly influences our shared mental health. This relational dimension of mental

health highlights the importance of community, hospitality, and acceptance in creating spaces where individuals can flourish.

(3) *Peace with Creation:* Creation is the space in the universe that God has given God's creatures responsibility for and to which God has asked them to offer care and tenderness (Gen 2:15). Tending for creation involves paying attention to ecological issues. The ground on which we stand matters. Tending and caring for creation also means paying proper attention to cultural, political, and economic matters. As will become clear, there is a close connection among how we structure the world, how we choose to behave toward creation, and our mental health. Disharmony within creation inevitably brings about disharmony within individuals and communities. We cannot understand one without the other.[10]

(4) *Peace with God:* Peace with God serves as the all-encompassing focus and desire of faithful mental healthcare. Living peaceably with God is the driving vision that shapes and forms all Christian mental healthcare practices.

CONCLUSION

Thinking of shalom as mental health provides us with a comprehensive perspective on the multifaceted

[10] The interplay between ecological health and mental health is increasingly evident in both scientific research

nature of mental healthcare. It encompasses care of

---

and lived experience. For instance, studies have shown that access to green spaces or natural settings positively impacts mental well-being, reducing stress, improving mood, and fostering resilience. Practices like "forest bathing" or spending intentional time in nature are now recognized as therapeutic, offering both physiological and psychological benefits. On the other hand, environmental degradation, displacement due to ecological crises, and the existential threat of climate change have all been linked to rising mental health concerns, including anxiety, depression, and a pervasive sense of hopelessness, often referred to as "climate anxiety." Beyond ecological considerations, the broader systems that shape our lives—political, economic, and cultural—are deeply interconnected with mental health. Inequitable economic systems, for example, exacerbate stress through financial insecurity, poor housing, and lack of access to basic resources. Political systems that marginalize or oppress contribute to a sense of alienation and powerlessness, eroding mental well-being. Conversely, systems that promote justice, equity, and cultural preservation provide a foundation for shalom, nurturing both personal and communal flourishing. Practical responses that align with this vision of shalom are already emerging in various contexts. Initiatives such as ecotherapy or nature-based mental health interventions tap into the healing power of creation, fostering deeper connections with the natural world as a pathway to healing. Community gardening projects, which bring people together to tend the earth while fostering relationships, offer similar benefits. At a systemic level, policies aimed at ensuring economic stability—through living wages, affordable housing, and universal access to healthcare—can significantly reduce the mental health burdens caused by individual minds, nurturing relationships between minds, stewardship of creation, and cultivating a

---

systemic injustice. Cultural and political engagement also play a vital role. For example, preserving cultural traditions and practices among Indigenous or marginalized groups nurtures identity and belonging, essential for mental well-being. Similarly, encouraging faith communities to advocate for justice-oriented policies, such as equitable resource distribution or robust climate action, embodies the kind of communal responsibility to creation that Gen 2:15 invites. Ultimately, the harmony we seek in creation is inseparable from the harmony we seek within ourselves and our communities. By tending to creation—ecologically, politically, and culturally—we participate in the unfolding of shalom. These acts, however small, provide glimpses of God's kingdom breaking into the present, affirming the hope that shalom is possible even in a fractured world. See Susan Clayton and Christie Manning, "Mental Health and Our Changing Climate: Impacts, Implications, and Guidance," American Psychological Association and EcoAmerica, 2017, https://www.apa.org/news/press/releases/2017/03/mental-health-climate.pdf; Kirsten Hayes and Neville Ellis, "Climate Change and Mental Health: Risks, Impacts and Priority Actions," *International Journal of Mental Health Systems* 12 (2018): 28, https://doi.org/10.1186/s13033-018-0210-6; Stephen Kaplan, "The Restorative Benefits of Nature: Toward an Integrative Framework," *Journal of Environmental Psychology* 15, no. 3 (1995): 169–82, https://doi.org/10.1016/0272-4944(95)90001-2; Mayo Clinic, "The Mental Health Benefits of Nature: Spending Time Outdoors to Refresh Your Mind," Mayo Clinic Press, 2024, https://mcpress.mayoclinic.org/mental-health/the-mental-health-benefits-of-nature-spending-time-outdoors-to-refresh-your-mind/.

tender and compassionate connection with God. Each of these dimensions is essential for a holistic approach to mental healthcare that is faithful to the practices of shalom. To honor the essence of faithful mental healthcare, we must consider each of these aspects with fidelity and intent. In the following chapters, we will explore each dimension, seeking to understand how they interweave to create a rich tapestry that enables the pursuit of faith-filled holistic mental healthcare.

2
PEACE WITHIN MINDS REQUIRES PEACE BETWEEN MINDS

Why the Inner Life Is Always Already Relational

I have suggested that *shalom relates to peace both within and between minds*. This statement raises the important question of what the mind is and where it resides. The inquiry into what the mind is and its location is not merely a philosophical curiosity; it shapes how we understand human identity, agency, and mental well-being. When reflecting on the mind, many of us might gesture toward our heads. However, there are other ways and places we can identify the mind. So, *what do we mean when we speak of "the mind?"*

The theory of mind that has been particularly influential in the West suggests that the mind is generated by the brain and is therefore primarily located within individual craniums, bounded by skin and skull. Here, the mind is considered an internal, private, and personal entity belonging to discrete individuals. Within this framework, mental ill-health is described in terms of *personal* disorders, which consequently affect private, isolated bodies containing minds that exist separately from those of others. We reflect this individualization of the mind in the responses we have developed to assist people in psychological distress. Many of our primary methods for addressing psychological distress—counseling, psychotherapy, cognitive behavioral therapy, and psychopharmacology—assume the existence of distinct minds that require therapeutic interventions to alleviate individual mental struggles.

EXPANDING OUR MINDS

Without diminishing the significance of therapeutic and pharmacological interventions aimed at individual minds (as we have seen, peace within minds is significant), it is important to note that such practices arise from and reflect a specific culture's understanding of the mind. The individualization of minds parallels the individualistic assumptions of Western culture. By individualism I refer to a value system and worldview that emphasizes the primacy of human freedom and autonomy over community and dependency. Freedom and autonomy are regarded as rights for everyone and are embedded in social, political, economic, and religious structures. As free, morally equal beings, individuals bear no formal responsibility towards others, other than to ensure that the exercise of their freedom and autonomy does not infringe upon the freedom and autonomy of others. In this perspective, the notion that minds are individual entities owned by single individuals, who bear primary responsibility for them without needing to reference other minds, appears evident. However, the dominant theory of mind in the West is in fact a minority viewpoint compared to other nations and cultures. Other cultures with alternative theories of mind employ different forms of intervention. Journalist and mental health commentator Brent Watters notes that not recognizing this cultural difference becomes problematic when we attempt to export therapeutic concepts from individualistic cultures to collective cultures. Taking Western mental health modes of intervention underpinned by a Western theory of mind can lead to the imposition of practices that are culturally inappropriate and potentially damaging.[1]

Mind and culture

Ideas about the mind then differ, sometimes quite significantly, across cultures. Anthropologists have

[1] Ethan Watters, *Crazy Like Us* (Robinson, 2011). Watters argues that mental illnesses are not universal but

long demonstrated that cultural contexts generate different ways of understanding thought, emotion, and selfhood. What one society might call an individual's "inner world" may be seen as something fundamentally shared, distributed, or even open to spiritual influence in another culture. These differences are not simply matters of linguistic preference; they shape how people experience and interpret the world around them. The anthropologist Tanya Luhrmann puts it this way:

> There is something phenomenologically basic about the human experience of awareness, or consciousness. All ethnographies describe people who think, feel, imagine, hope, and are aware. Yet anthropologists have shown that different social worlds understand mental life (we will call this "mind") in different ways. Different cultures imagine mental life differently, both in what thought can do, and how one might draw the boundary between mind and world. These culturally different understandings have real social consequences. They affect the way that people imagine what it is to be a self, the way

are shaped by cultural beliefs. As American views about mental health spread globally, they are changing how other cultures understand and express mental ill-health.

> they understand time and history, the way they understand spirits and rituals, the way they experience illness and health.[2]

The way we conceptualize the mind has profound implications for our understanding and practical engagement with the world.

Local theories of mind

Luhrmann describes these different ways of understanding the mind as "local theories of mind."[3] For example, in Melanesian and South Pacific societies one often encounters what anthropologists call the *opacity of mind theory*. In these cultural contexts it is not assumed that individuals have direct access to one another's thoughts, nor is it considered appropriate to infer someone's inner intentions unless they explicitly state them. Social life is structured around verbalized statements rather than presumed mental states. In contrast, Western societies tend to assume the transparency of mind—that is, we believe that people's inner motivations can be

[2] Tanya Marie Luhrmann, "Mind," in *The Open Encyclopedia of Anthropology*, ed. Felix Stein, facsimile of the 1st ed. in *The Cambridge Encyclopedia of Anthropology* (Cambridge University Press, 2023 [2021]), http://doi.org/10.29164/21mind.

[3] Luhrmann, "Mind," 7.

read through body language, facial expressions, or subtle cues.[4] These assumptions govern everything from legal systems to psychological therapy, yet they are not universal.

Other societies embrace porous theories of mind, where the boundaries between personal thought, the social world, and even the spiritual realm are much more fluid. For example, among certain Indigenous communities, cognition is viewed as coextensive with the environment, meaning that interactions with land, ritual, and communal memory dynamically shape one's thinking. In this context, the mind is not merely housed in the brain but extends across social and spiritual spaces, intertwined with relational and sacred realities.

The Western theory of mind I have described above is just as local. Luhrmann points out that "this sense of mind as a thing, as the seat of the self, as the driver of action, as something inner which is separate from an outer world; these are Western preoccupations, not Kwakiutl, Canaque, or Dinka preoccupations."[5] Similarly, the identification of mind with personal identity—"I am what I think I am"—is culturally specific. Indigenous people, for example,

[4] Luhrmann, "Mind," 7.
[5] Luhrmann, "Mind," 5.

see mind and memory as residing in the land, in stories, in song, and within communities.[6]

If we are to engage in effective mental healthcare that takes cultural diversity seriously, recognizing the contextual nature of our theory of mind is vital. This is not to suggest that we should entirely reject the Western concept of mind; however, we must acknowledge its limitations and refine our understanding by considering alternative perspectives—one of which, as will become clear, is the perspective we find in the Bible. However, before we explore this, there is more to be said about the nature of the mind.

These anthropological perspectives challenge the Western tendency to view cognition as a solitary event occurring solely within individual minds. Instead, they propose a model in which the mind is socially distributed, environmentally extended, and fundamentally relational. This perspective has significant implications for mental health. If mental well-being is not merely about individual brain function but is also shaped by the quality of relationships, community stability, and environmental

[6] Michelle R. Jacobs, *Indigenous Memory, Urban Reality: Stories of American Indian Relocation and Reclamation* (New York University Press, 2023).

structure, then healing must extend beyond the individual and into shared spaces of meaning, connection, and support.

"THE WESTERN MIND"?

Thus far, I have discussed the Western mind as if there were only one theory of mind in the West. It is indeed true that assumptions about the individualized mind are central, either implicitly or explicitly, to much of our thinking about and responding to mental health. Nevertheless, there are other significant ways in which the mind is conceptualized in the West. Here, we will examine two perspectives that are particularly relevant to both mental health/shalom and a theology of the mind: *Extended Mind Theory* and *Interpersonal Neurobiology*. Each of these perspectives on the mind challenges the notion of the individual mind and offers important insights into the idea that the brain is fundamentally shaped by attachment, emotion, and social engagement. They also provide the groundwork for a practical and theological understanding of "the mind of Christ," which has important implications for our developing understanding of shalomic mental health.

Extended Mind Theory

In their 1998 paper "The Extended Mind,"[7] philosophers Andy Clark and David Chalmers ask: "Where does mind stop and the rest of the world begin?"[8] They suggest there are two standard replies.

> Some accept the boundaries of skin and skull and say that what is outside the body is outside the mind. Others are impressed by arguments suggesting that the meaning of our words "just ain't in the head," and hold that this externalism about meaning carries over into an externalism about mind.[9]

They suggest a third position, a quite different kind of externalism: "an *active externalism*, based on the active role of the environment in driving cognitive processes."[10] This is a radical idea: *cognition does not stop at the brain's boundaries.*[11] The suggestion is that objects outside of the brain, such as pens, paper, or

[7] Andy Clark and David Chalmers, "The Extended Mind," *Analysis* 58, no. 1 (1998): 7–19.

[8] Clark and Chalmers, "Extended Mind," 7.

[9] Clark and Chalmers, "Extended Mind," 7.

[10] Clark and Chalmers, "Extended Mind," 7.

[11] Radical for Westerners, but less so for Indigenous people, as mentioned previously.

phones, perform similar functions to parts of the brain. In their now-famous example, they describe a man named Otto, who has early-stage Alzheimer's. Otto relies on a notebook to remember key information—addresses, names, and daily tasks. Rather than treating the notebook as a mere tool, Clark and Chalmers argue that it acts as an extension of Otto's cognitive process.[12] In effect, his mind is not simply in his brain but distributed throughout the world. This theory—Extended Mind Theory (EMT)—suggests that we should not think of cognition as something that occurs solely inside the head. Rather, mental processes depend on external scaffolding.

Cognitive scaffolding

By *scaffolding* Clark and Chalmers refer to external structures that support and enhance cognitive processes, reducing mental effort by offloading tasks onto the environment.[13] Minds are not sealed off from their environments; they rely on external supports. Tools, language, social rituals, embodied practices, and, increasingly, social media and mobile phones extend cognition into the world. In a

[12] Clark and Chalmers, "Extended Mind," 12.

[13] Andy Clark, *Being There: Putting Brain, Body and World Together Again* (MIT Press, 1997).

spiritual context, we might envision someone using a prayer book to guide meditation. When people implement such conduits, they are not merely referencing an external source but offloading part of their cognitive burden onto a structured external system that supports and directs their thoughts. The Eucharist and communal lament serve a similar function by externalizing the emotional and cognitive work of remembering, processing grief, and shaping spiritual consciousness.

Socially distributed cognition

This way of thinking changes our understanding of cognition. People do not merely think in isolation; they think *with* and *through* others and via other objects in the world. Conversations, collective worship, storytelling, and shared decision-making function as extensions of individual cognition. This is an important point. If we accept that minds are interwoven with community, mental well-being cannot be separated from relational networks. A person struggling with anxiety or depression may not need only internal therapeutic interventions (although these are, of course, still important); they may need a transformation in their social world—reconnection to communal practices, friendships, and embodied rituals that extend their cognitive capacity.

The kind of creatures we are

These insights challenge the hegemony of Western models of mental health, which focus solely on *fixing internal states* instead of *modifying external environments and social networks*. EMT also offers insight into the nature of healing. Healing in this context is not just about correcting faulty neurochemistry or reframing thoughts (though it does not, of course, exclude these aspects); it involves reshaping the cognitive scaffolding that individuals rely on for meaning, memory, and emotional regulation.

It is worth noting that EMT is not necessarily a factual claim.[14] One could make a strong case for

[14] The distinction between a factual claim and a conceptual framework is important in understanding Extended Mind Theory. A factual claim is one that can be tested empirically, such as whether cognitive processes measurably extend into external tools like notebooks or smartphones. However, EMT is better understood as a philosophical perspective on cognition rather than a strictly empirical hypothesis. It challenges the notion of the mind as self-contained, instead proposing that human thought is inherently relational and embedded in the world. This perspective resonates with the kind of theological understandings of human interdependence that emerge from the concept of shalom, which emphasizes peace, justice, and the interconnectedness of persons within their environment, ideas developed more fully later in this chapter. While some aspects of EMT may be supported by cognitive science,

both sides. As MacFarquhar, writing in the *New Yorker*, puts it:

> . . . more a way of thinking about what sort of creature a human is. Clark rejects the idea that a person is complete in himself [sic], shut in against the outside, in no need of help.[15]

We are relational, embodied creatures whose corporate nature is not limited by the boundaries of our bodies but extends into creation in ways that resonate closely with our previous reflections on shalom. Peace within and between minds has a vital environmental dimension that is deeply connected to shalom's insistence that justice is necessary for health. MacFarquhar puts it this way:

> If a person's thought was intimately linked to her surroundings, then destroying a person's surroundings could be as damaging and reprehensible as a bodily attack. If certain kinds of

---

its broader implications extend into philosophy, ethics, and theology, making it less a matter of factual verification and more a way of reimagining the nature of human cognition.

[15] Larissa MacFarquhar, "The Mind-Expanding Ideas of Andy Clark," *New Yorker*, March 26, 2018.

> thought required devices like paper and pens, then the kind of poverty that precluded them looked as debilitating as a brain lesion. Moreover, by emphasizing how thoroughly everyone was dependent on the structure of his or her world, it showed how disabled people who were dependent on things like ramps were no different from anybody else. Some theorists had argued that disability was often a feature less of a person than of a built environment that failed to take some needs into account; the extended-mind thesis showed how clearly this was so.[16]

We do not have space to explore this intriguing idea of what we might call "mind poverty." However, we will touch on related issues when we explore

[16] MacFarquhar, "Mind-Expanding Ideas." Although we can't draw them out in detail here, the implications of EMT for disability theology are significant. If cognition is not confined to the brain but extends into the environment, then disabling barriers—whether physical, social, or technological—are not just inconveniences but direct impediments to thought and agency. This aligns with the social model of disability, which emphasizes that disability is not merely a personal limitation but a result of environmental failures to accommodate diverse needs. See Tom Shakespeare, *Disability Rights and Wrongs Revisited* (Routledge, 2013). EMT reinforces the theological claim that human flourishing is relational and dependent

neoliberalism and environmental destruction later in this book. For now, the key thing to notice is that *shalomic mental health expands beyond the brain.*

Interpersonal Neurobiology

This revised philosophical way of thinking about the mind finds empirical resonance within the field of *Interpersonal Neurobiology* (IPNB). Developed by Daniel Siegal,[17] Allan Schore,[18] and others,[19] IPNB argues that the brain is fundamentally shaped by attachment, emotion, and social engagement. This field expands the idea that minds are not only extended beyond individuals but are also *emergent properties of and between individuals*

on justice, hospitality, and the removal of structural exclusions—central themes in disability theology.

[17] Daniel J. Siegel, *The Developing Mind: Toward a Neurobiology of Interpersonal Experience* (Guilford Press, 1999); 3rd ed., *The Developing Mind: How Relationships and the Brain Interact to Shape Who We Are* (Guilford Press, 2020).

[18] Allan Schore, "The Interpersonal Neurobiology of Intersubjectivity," *Frontiers in Psychology* 12 (2021).

[19] In particular, Curt Thompson has used this approach in his theological reflections on the importance of relationships and being known: Curt Thompson, *Anatomy of the Soul: Surprising Connections Between Neuroscience and Spiritual Practices That Can Transform Your Life and Relationships* (Tyndale Refresh, 2010).

through relationships.[20] Unlike neuroreductionist approaches[21] that reduce mental activity to neural mechanisms, and unlike Extended Mind Theory, which emphasizes functional cognitive extensions, IPNB presents the mind as an emergent property of social and interpersonal processes.

At its core, IPNB rejects the concept of a self-contained mind, arguing instead that cognition, emotional regulation, and even biological processes are inherently coregulated and co-constructed within *relationships*. Rather than emphasizing internal representational processing, as per traditional cognitive science models, IPNB highlights the affective, embodied, and intersubjective nature of mental life. The mind does not exist solely *within* the individual; it emerges *between* people, distributed across

[20] Daniel J. Siegel and Chloe Drulis, "An Interpersonal Neurobiology Perspective on the Mind and Mental Health: Personal, Public, and Planetary Well-Being," *Annals of General Psychiatry* 22, no. 1 (2023): 5, https://annals-general-psychiatry.biomedcentral.com/articles/10.1186/s12991-023-00434-5.

[21] A dominant strand in cognitive neuroscience has been neuroreductionism, the view that mental states are fully explicable in terms of neural activity and brain function. This paradigm has reinforced biomedical approaches to mental health, which conceptualize psychological disorders as individual neurochemical imbalances rather than relational dysfunctions.

relational systems, emerging through patterns of connection and mutual regulation.

In addition to encouraging us to consider the significance of viewing the mind in relational terms (peace between minds), this perspective has profound implications for understanding mental health and mental healthcare. If cognition and emotional regulation are inherently relational, therapeutic interventions must address the individual and the wider relational and social systems that foster well-being. Importantly, recognizing the mind as a coregulated, affectively mediated, and intersubjectively embedded phenomenon challenges traditional Western concepts of autonomy and selfhood, directing attention instead to a model of human flourishing rooted in relational integrity, attunement, and connection.[22]

[22] This has important implications, for example, for people with advanced dementia in that it challenges dominant paradigms of cognition, autonomy, and selfhood. If cognition and emotional regulation are inherently relational, then dementia cannot be understood solely as an individual neurological decline but must also be examined in relation to the social and relational environments in which a person is embedded. This perspective suggests that personhood is not lost with cognitive deterioration but is instead co-constituted by relationships, emotional attunement, and embodied presence. It highlights the importance of relational attunement in caregiving, where nonverbal communication, sensory engagement, and affective connection remain central

Mental health: To the brain and beyond!

Interpersonal Neurobiology converges with Anthropology and Extended Mind Theory in asserting that minds are fundamentally relational. Our environment beyond our bodies is significant for peace of mind and harmony between minds; this does not occur solely through introspection but rather through external changes in relationships, community, and participation in rituals. The presence of others—attuned, listening, and physically present—rewires neural pathways, reinforcing resilience and emotional well-being. By integrating insights from anthropology, EMT, and IPNB we come to understand the mind as:

- *Socially Situated:* Minds are shaped by culture and relationships, not just by individual biology.
- *Extended Beyond the Body:* Cognition is distributed across tools, communities, and external environments.
- *Relationally Emergent:* Healing depends not just on internal change but on attachment, shared rituals, and communal care.

---

to well-being. Furthermore, it challenges the traditional medical model of dementia care by underscoring the need to focus not only on the individual but also on the relational and communal structures that support flourishing. Theologically, this shifts the emphasis from autonomy to relational integrity, reinforcing a vision of human flourishing rooted in connectedness, presence, and dignity rather than cognitive ability.

Instead of viewing mental health as a private matter, this model encourages us to examine the systems, relationships, and external structures that influence human flourishing. If minds extend beyond brains, then healing should not be limited to individuals, it should be pursued collectively, within minds, between minds, and in connection with the broader dimensions of creation.

THE BODY AND MIND OF CHRIST: BEYOND METAPHOR

Turning now to theology, we can begin to see how these insights from anthropology, EMT, and IPNB help us understand and ground certain key theological ideas about the mind. Within Scripture, body, mind, and soul are inextricably interconnected; what occurs in one domain is mirrored in the others.[23] To understand the mind, we must also comprehend the body. New Testament scholar Susan Eastman, in her reflections on the apostle Paul's perspective on personhood, points out that for Paul human beings are not viewed as *monological* individuals. Rather, they are understood as inherently *dialogical creatures*. This is evident from the moment of creation, where the writer of

[23] Michael J. Boivin, "The Hebraic Model of the Person: Toward a Unified Psychological Science Among Christian Helping Professionals," *Journal of Psychology and Theology* 19, no. 2 (1991): 157–65.

Genesis tells us that we are made to be with others; it is not good for us to be alone (Gen 2:18). Human beings are contingent and interdependent creatures designed to live in harmonious, dialogical relationships with one another and with God. Human flourishing, Eastman insists, arises when we exist in a state of *participation and belonging*.[24] As we engage in one another's lives, we experience a sense of belonging, a feeling of being at home in the world. This sense of belonging is personal, but it also exists *between* individuals and larger social bodies, such as political and economic systems, religions, and other powers and principalities.[25] As we saw in chapter 1, participation and belonging are indicators of the presence of shalom. Thus far in this chapter we have illustrated why this is significant at both a philosophical and neurological level. This aligns with our understanding as creatures made in the image of a triune, relational God who, by taking bodily form in the life and death of

[24] Susan G. Eastman, "Bodies, Agency, and the Relational Self: A Pauline Approach to the Goals and Use of Psychiatric Drugs," *Christian Bioethics: Non-Ecumenical Studies in Medical Morality* 24, no. 3 (2018): 288–301, doi:10.1093/CB/CBY011.

[25] Eastman, "Bodies, Agency, and the Relational Self," 288.

Jesus, underscores the importance of bodies for our journey with God and one another.

In a beautifully poetic turn, Eastman informs us that for Paul "it is as if physical bodies were *bridges* rather than *barriers*, making human creatures into participatory beings, not autonomous, not isolated, but connected to larger 'bodies.'"[26] In this understanding, we have independent bodies and minds, but they are situated in the world differently than the kind of individualism highlighted previously. We are simultaneously *independent*—others do not swallow up our identity; we remain ourselves; interdependent—our actions occur in partnerships of mutuality with others; and yet also *dependent—entirely* reliant on God. Individuality and corporeality are tied together in *noncompetitive bonds of love*. It is not as *I* flourish that *I* find well-being, but as *we* flourish that *we* find well-being (shalom) *together* (1 Cor 12:26). Similar to the theological model of health and well-being laid out in chapter 1 and the integrated model of extended mind presented earlier in this chapter, human flourishing is never a solitary enterprise. This noncompetitive relationality is crucial to bear

[26] Eastman, "Bodies, Agency, and the Relational Self," 292.

in mind, especially in relation to the discussion we will have in chapter 3 regarding individuality, neoliberalism, and the market economy.

This deep relationality is a blessing that also makes us profoundly physically and psychologically vulnerable. When we are neglected, abused, ignored, or traumatized, these experiences inevitably impede our flourishing, as they push against the essence of who and what we are as contingent relational creatures. God intended us to exist "in the mode of belonging."[27] We suffer when that intention is frustrated by negative individual or social experiences. The reality that much of our psychological suffering arises from the damage and fragmentation of our natural, God-given desire to relate, participate, and belong—whether as children or as we navigate the world as adults—adds a theological poignancy to the significance of Paul's model of persons. *People need therapy and medication, but above all else, they need and desire love, acceptance, and a sense of belonging.*

PAUL AND THE MIND OF CHRIST

The relationality and interconnectivity of our bodies—our embodied desire for shalom—are reflected in the interconnective dynamics that

[27] Eastman, "Bodies, Agency, and the Relational Self," 299.

comprise our minds. For Paul, our minds are also inherently dialogical and, as such, inevitably vulnerable.

Toward a Christian theory of mind

In light of what has been discussed thus far, it is interesting to note that Christians tend to have at least two theories of mind.[28] Christians often share the Westernized theory of mind that sees the mind as an intracranial phenomenon. They are as likely as anyone else to locate the mind in the individual head and act accordingly. Simultaneously, however, they adhere to a very different theory of mind. They oscillate between a localized Western theory of mind and a significant innovation that challenges and contradicts that view. Christians assume the mind is a closed, personal entity. They generally do not consider hearing strange voices in their heads a normal or desirable experience. Yet at the same time they accept that God can put thoughts and words into

[28] By this, I am not referring to double-mindedness, a state of inner conflict where a person is torn between faithfulness to God and worldly desires, leading to instability in thought and action, as per, for example, Jas 1:8: "For the doubter, being double-minded and unstable in every way . . ." (NRSV). This verse is part of a passage that explains that believers should believe in God and not doubt.

their minds. Through spiritual practices—prayer, meditation, Scripture reading—we can work to discern which thoughts are ours and which come from God.[29] Thoughts and experiences given by God from outside our minds carry practical implications. One hears a word from God in one's mind and then acts according to what that voice says. More troubling is the tendency to equate unusual experiences, such as hearing voices, with demonic forces influencing the mind. Positively and negatively, for Christians the mind is porous and permeable at the levels of the divine and the demonic.[30] However, this apparent tension between enclosedness and porosity/permeability is eased if we reflect on the theory of mind the apostle Paul held in relation to both human minds and, importantly, the mind of Christ.

Sharing in the mind of Christ

New Testament scholar Paula Gooder, in her reflections on Paul's view of the mind, informs us that there is a dynamic corporality to Paul's understanding, which is revealed not only in the body, as per

[29] For further development of the nature of this process see T. M. Luhrmann, *When God Talks Back: Understanding the American Evangelical Relationship with God* (Knopf, 2012).

[30] Chris Cook, *Hearing Voices Demonic and Divine: Scientific and Theological Perspectives* (Routledge, 2020).

Eastman, but also in his concept of mind.[31] According to Paul, and in line with the theoretical perspectives we have developed thus far, we do not merely possess isolated individual minds; instead, our minds participate in a larger, relational reality—the mind of Christ. This participation is not reducible to biological or psychological processes alone but is mediated through the body of Christ (1 Cor 12:12) and the indwelling presence of the Holy Spirit, who unites us with the mind of Christ (1 Cor 2:15–16). In this way, cognition, perception, and transformation are not solely functions of neural activity or social interaction but are also shaped by the Spirit, drawing us into the very life and wisdom of Jesus.

The mind of Christ

In 1 Corinthians 2:15–16 Paul states, "The person with the Spirit makes judgments about all things, but such a person is not subject to merely human judgments; for, 'Who has known the mind of the Lord so as to instruct him?' But we have the mind of Christ" (NIV). Before Jesus came, humans couldn't understand what God thought; but now, in Jesus and

[31] Paula Gooder, "Paul, the Mind and the Mind of Christ," in *The Bible and Mental Health: Towards a Biblical Theology of Mental Health*, ed. Chris Cook, Isabelle Hamley, and Justin Welby (SCM, 2020), 74–83.

through the Spirit, our minds are transformed (Rom 12:2) and extended in such a way that we can share in the mind of Christ and be changed as we come to comprehend what was previously incomprehensible. Why was it previously incomprehensible? Because without Jesus, we were unable to think the way we do now, that we can share in the mind of Christ.[32] At a very fundamental level, sharing in the mind of Christ renews our minds[33] and enables us to think thoughts we could never conceive alone.

Gooder points out a subtle nuance in Philippians 2:5: "In your relationships with one another, have

[32] This reminds us of Extended Mind Theory's assertion that without external input we cannot think in certain ways. Before Jesus, human minds lacked the cognitive framework to grasp divine wisdom. The incarnation of Jesus and the presence of the Spirit function as external cognitive scaffolds, enabling a new mode of thought—one that allows participation in the "mind of Christ." Without this external extension, divine comprehension would remain inaccessible, just as complex reasoning (like mathematical thinking) is impossible without prior exposure to its external structures.

[33] Central to the conversation in this chapter is that the concept of *neuroplasticity*—the brain's ability to reorganize and form new neural connections in response to experience—closely aligns with the idea that sharing in the mind of Christ renews our minds. Just as new experiences, relationships, and learning reshape neural pathways, participation in the mind of Christ through

the same mindset as Christ Jesus" (NIV). This verse encourages us to adopt Christ's way of thinking collectively, particularly in how we relate to one another. Once again, this nuance challenges the notion that our minds are purely private and personal. The anthropological, philosophical, and neurological theories we explored earlier suggest that while each of us possesses internal mental mechanisms unique to ourselves, sharing in the mind of Christ invites us to extend our thoughts outward. In doing so, we are transformed—our minds are renewed. Sharing in the mind of Christ is not merely about acquiring

---

the Spirit fundamentally transforms cognitive patterns, enabling believers to think in ways previously impossible. Neuroplasticity entails that repeated exposure to new ways of thinking and acting physically changes the brain, making new patterns of thought and behavior more natural over time. Similarly, Paul's claim that we are "transformed by the renewing of our minds" (Rom 12:2) suggests that immersion in the life of Christ reconfigures human cognition, allowing believers to perceive, judge, and act in alignment with divine wisdom, rather than being limited by prior mental frameworks. Thus, just as neuroplasticity enables intellectual and behavioral transformation through sustained interaction with external stimuli, the "mind of Christ" serves as a divine cognitive scaffold that reshapes human thought through spiritual participation. Cf. Norman Doidge, *The Brain That Changes Itself: Stories of Personal Triumph from the Frontiers of Brain Science* (Viking Press, 2007).

knowledge of Jesus; it is about learning to think collectively and recognizing the power of relationships to shape our thinking, externalizing our thoughts in ways that align with the one who embodies shalom.

Embodied minds

Our minds' reciprocal and relational nature can either foster a virtuous cycle of growth and healing or create a destructive cycle of harm and distortion. The shared mind of Christ, when faithfully stewarded, serves as a source of healing and unity; however, it is susceptible to corruption when misused or misapplied.[34] Engaging in collective thinking

[34] When misapplied, the concept of the shared mind of Christ can enable spiritual abuse by fostering authoritarian control, theological distortion, and exclusion. Leaders who claim exclusive access to divine wisdom may demand unquestioning obedience, suppressing individual discernment. Harmful theological interpretations can justify suffering or stigmatize mental illness as a spiritual failure rather than addressing systemic or psychological realities. In some cases, gaslighting occurs when individuals are led to believe their doubts or pain result from weak faith, causing self-blame and psychological harm. Additionally, rigid interpretations of Christian unity can lead to sectarianism and exclusion, where those who think differently are marginalized rather than embraced. Properly stewarding the mind of Christ requires discernment to prevent its misuse as a tool of control rather than a source of healing and transformation.

that aligns with Christ's values allows us to cultivate wholeness and restoration. Conversely, harmful patterns of thought within communities can lead to severe consequences, such as spiritual abuse, alienation, stigma, and theological distortion. For example, attributing mental health struggles to personal sin, labeling psychosis as the work of demonic forces, or questioning the salvation of people with dementia because they have forgotten who Jesus is illustrates how misguided shared thinking can inflict harm. Such errors wound individuals and reshape communal minds in ways that perpetuate suffering rather than alleviate it. Recognizing that we actively shape, nurture, and influence one another's minds underscores the moral responsibility of stewarding the individual and corporate mind with care. This is not simply an ethical duty but a fundamental aspect of faithful mental healthcare. Later in this book, we will explore how neglecting cultural context can undermine mental well-being. Likewise, failing to recognize dangerous flaws in collective thought can lead to deeply harmful practices that reinforce stigma, alienation, and spiritual harm.

Three dimensions of mind

To sum up our reflections on the mind, the Christian mind can be understood as the intertwining of three intricately connected dimensions: the mind within the skull, the extended mind as it engages with others, and the mind as it participates in the mind of Christ. Resonating with Eastman's observations about the dialogical nature of the body, Christian minds are also shared and dialogical. Descartes's dictum, "I think therefore I am," which has greatly influenced ideas about Western identity and the Western mind, comes under serious scrutiny when we recognize the implications of sharing in the corporate mind of Christ. As Gooder puts it:

> Paul's theology—and in particular his references to having the mind of Christ—suggests that there is a corporate strand to the mind that our modern culture often overlooks. Thinking, feeling and imagining together as the body of Christ inspired by the Spirit can shape our minds so that we think and act like Christ, seeing the world as Christ did.[35]

THE IMPORTANCE OF THE CORPORATE MIND OF CHRIST

Why is it important to reflect on the shared and porous nature of the mind in the context of mental health

[35] Gooder, "Paul and the Mind of Christ," 78.

and mental healthcare? First of all, understanding the interconnection of our minds compels us to take responsibility not only for our own thoughts but also for the impact our words, actions, and presence have on the minds of others. Recognizing that our bodies and minds are shared and shaped through dialogue and community heightens our awareness of the need to keep the fruits of the Spirit at the forefront of our thoughts and actions (Gal 5:22–26). Living lives marked by gentleness, kindness, patience, and love, striving to avoid careless talk, controlling our tongues (Jas 3:1–2), and acknowledging the formative power of words on the minds of others help us resist conforming to the patterns of this world. In this way, we embrace the corporate connectedness of our minds and bodies.

As Paul urges in Romans 12:2, "Do not conform to the pattern of this world, but be transformed by the renewing of your mind. Then you will be able to test and approve what God's will is, his good, pleasing and perfect will" (NIV). This transformation involves reshaping our minds in the light of Christ's mind. It is a corporate process that requires us to recognize how our minds interact with others and to take responsibility for disciplining our minds in ways that bring love and healing to the minds of our neighbors. Failing to act this way risks harming others' minds. Acknowledging the permeability and interconnection of bodies and minds calls us to love our neighbor's mind as we love our own. Recognizing the corporate dimensions of the mind is central to discipleship and foundational for faithful mental healthcare.

Secondly, adopting a corporate perspective on body and mind shifts our understanding of mental health challenges from a purely individualistic viewpoint. While individuals may encounter unique forms of psychological distress that require care, treatment, and attention, these challenges cannot be fully addressed in isolation. The work of mental health professionals with individuals is both vital and necessary; for some, medication plays an essential role in their treatment. Adjusting the chemistry of individual bodies can be a significant aspect of mental healthcare. However, focusing solely on the individual without considering their relationships and environments overlooks a critical dimension of mental health. As we will explore in chapter 3, it is essential to consider the question, "What is wrong with *you*?" alongside another equally important question: "What might be wrong with *us*?"

Third, on an emotional level, recognizing the corporeality and porosity of the human mind provides comfort when we feel, in some way, that we are "losing our minds." Conditions such as dementia or schizophrenia can profoundly alter one's personality, often leaving individuals feeling lost or disconnected from the person they once were. When our minds change, it is easy to assume that our very identity has also changed—sometimes to the point of becoming unrecognizable. If we believe our identity is solely tied to the inner workings of our minds, such changes can leave us feeling isolated and alienated from both ourselves and others.

Without diminishing the real pain of such experiences, the understanding that our minds are shared can offer a measure of reassurance. While we may feel we are changing, we still share in the mind of Christ, whose unchanging nature provides a steady foundation. When our own minds falter we can rest assured that Christ's mind remains constant and faithful towards us. Ideally, this constancy is reflected in the body of Christ—the church—which, through its shared participation in the corporate mind of Jesus, holds us in solidarity when we feel our minds "slipping away." Shared minds mean that none of us struggles alone: *the body and mind of Christ participate in each of our mental health challenges.*

THE DANGERS OF REDUCTIONISM?

It is not unreasonable to ask whether the interdisciplinary engagement I have pursued—drawing from anthropology, EMT, and IPNB—risks a form of theological reductionism. Might integrating empirical and philosophical perspectives into theology diminish or distort theological truths by assimilating them into frameworks shaped by fundamentally different epistemologies and ontologies?

This is a serious and valid concern. However, this work does not begin with scientific or philosophical insights and then seek to baptize them into theological meaning. Rather, it begins with the theological conviction that in Jesus Christ we see not only true divinity but also true humanity. To speak of "the mind" in Christian terms is to begin with the mind of Christ (1 Cor 2:16), a reality into which we are drawn through the Spirit's uniting work. This theological anthropology, rooted in participation, communion, and eschatological hope, serves as the interpretive lens through which all other insights must be critically assessed and re-narrated.

Within this framework, the contributions of disciplines such as EMT and IPNB are not constitutive but illustrative: they offer limited, contingent accounts of human relationality that can, when rightly interpreted, echo more profound theological truths. Their descriptive claims about the socially distributed, environmentally scaffolded, and relationally emergent nature of cognition resonate with what theology has long affirmed: that human beings are created for communion, not isolation; that our flourishing is bound to others, to creation, and to God. This is not to say that interdisciplinary dialogue carries no risk. Indeed, where theological categories are subordinated to scientific models or the canons of empirical verification judge theological claims, a reductive materialism can easily take hold. But this need not be the case. When read within a theological grammar centered on Christ, EMT's claim that cognition is extended and scaffolded by practices and environments can be seen as a secular analogue to the ecclesial body's role in shaping the mind of Christ within us. Similarly, IPNB's empirical observation that minds are formed and transformed in attuned relational matrices may be read as a confirmation, though not a foundation, of the theological truth that human beings are inherently dialogical and dependent, bearing the image of the triune God.

Crucially, the theological claim that we share in the mind of Christ (Phil 2:5) cannot be reduced to psychological processes or social configurations. It is a pneumatological and eschatological reality, grounded in the Spirit's transformative work and oriented toward the renewal of all things in Christ. It transcends naturalistic categories not by rejecting them, but by reordering them within a Christological horizon. Theology neither denies the truths science can offer nor allows them to determine its claims. Instead, it draws these insights into its wider telos, reinterpreting them in light of the gospel.

This reframing guards against both dualism and reductionism. Rather than separating theological and empirical insights into unrelated domains or collapsing one into the other, it holds them in a dynamic and critical relationship. The mind is not merely a neurobiological mechanism, nor only a theological construct; it is a locus of communion and vulnerability, a site of divine participation and human formation. Its mystery cannot be exhausted by neuroscience, but neither should theology ignore what careful, critical science can uncover about the conditions in which minds flourish or suffer. Indeed, to acknowledge the relational, porous, and communal nature of the mind, as these interdisciplinary frameworks suggest, is to affirm a vision deeply consonant with the biblical understanding of shalom: a state of right relation with God, self, others, and creation.

This is not to say that EMT or IPNB provide a doctrine of shalom, but rather that they may in limited ways illuminate its contours when viewed through theological lenses. Thus, rather than engaging in reductionism, this project aims to enact a kind of Christological expansion: drawing other disciplines into the orbit of theological meaning, transfiguring their insights in the light of the One in whom all things hold together (Col 1:17). The relational nature of mind, then, is not a discovery of contemporary science but a rediscovery—one that, when rightly understood, testifies to the depth and breadth of the peace offered in Jesus. Peace, as the previous chapter argued, is not found in the solitary individual but in communal, embodied, and Spirit-infused belonging. It is not simply psychological equilibrium, but participation in the One who is our peace (Eph 2:14). To think theologically about the mind, then, is to begin with Jesus, and to end there also.

CONCLUSION

In this chapter we have explored the vital implications of recognizing the shared and porous nature of the human mind for mental healthcare. This understanding challenges the Western notion of the mind as an isolated, individual entity and invites us to embrace a more relational and dialogical view, rooted in Scripture and enriched by interdisciplinary and cross-cultural perspectives. Such a shift requires us to consider not only personal transformation but also the corporate responsibility we carry for caring for one another's minds within the body of Christ.

The mind of Christ presents a model of interconnectedness, where healing, unity, and love are nurtured through collective participation in God's shalom. However, this shared dynamic also carries the weight of accountability; our words, actions, and attitudes toward one another can either foster flourishing or perpetuate harm. When we embrace the corporate mind of Christ with humility and intentionality, we align ourselves with God's transformative purposes, becoming agents of healing and belonging for others. By recognizing the interdependence of minds, we move beyond the limitations of individualistic approaches to mental healthcare and begin to address the relational, systemic, and indeed creational dimensions of well-being. This broadened understanding not only honors the relational nature of humanity as God intended but also establishes a foundation for faithful, compassionate mental healthcare that reflects the heart of the gospel.

Having considered peace within and between minds, we now turn to the third dimension of shalom: *peace with creation.*

3
FINDING PEACE WITH CREATION

Culture, Systems, Politics, and the Land

The shared nature of our minds, as explored in the previous chapter, makes us vulnerable to harm from others. This harm may be direct, originating from destructive or coercive relationships, or indirect, arising from alienation due to stigma, misunderstanding, prejudice, or systemic injustice. Loving our neighbors' minds is a vital aspect of faithful mental healthcare. The porosity of our bodies and minds also exposes us to influences beyond our immediate relationships. What occurs within creation—the environment where our bodies and minds live, breathe, and find their being—profoundly impacts our mental health. Disharmony within creation inevitably leads to disharmony within individuals and communities. This chapter focuses on these dimensions of shalom and mental health, emphasizing our relationship with creation. It explores how neglecting the care of creation undermines our mental well-being.

DEFINING CREATION

When I talk about care for creation, I am not merely addressing ecological issues; although, as will become clear, such matters are a significant part of the mental health conversation. Creation, as I use the term here, encompasses the land beneath our feet, the air that fills our lungs, and the geographic spaces we carve out to live and love. Within these geographical areas, there are visible elements, such as the physical condition of the land, as well as invisible factors like politics, economics, and culture. By creation, I refer to all of these dimensions. A lack of shalom in any of these areas leads to dissonance, instability, and mental ill-health. As I begin to explore the issues, I want to revisit the question posed in chapter 1: *What is mental health?* But this time from a different perspective. My starting point here is the rather unusual proposition that *a focus on mental health can be detrimental to our mental health.*

A FOCUS ON MENTAL HEALTH CAN BE BAD FOR OUR MENTAL HEALTH

Recently, there has been a commendable shift away from discussing mental health issues solely in terms of mental illness. Some individuals, particularly those who utilize mental health services, have argued that the term "illness" unnecessarily confines people within a medical framework and distinguishes them in the ways discussed in chapter 1. When this occurs, the assumption is that (a) some people are perpetually ill and (b) mental health problems should be addressed exclusively by mental health professionals. I don't mean to imply that we should avoid seeking professional care; I simply wish to emphasize that this is not the only way to frame or address people's experiences.

The term *mental illness* suggests that treatment and recovery primarily focus on eliminating symptoms. In contrast, advocates for framing experiences in terms of *mental health* argue that this approach offers a more positive and holistic perspective. It promotes a view of recovery that is not strictly tied to medical criteria but instead emphasizes enabling individuals to live in ways that align with their life goals and priorities. This approach allows people to find meaning and fulfillment, even amid experiences that others might perceive as unhealthy. In this sense, *mental health* can be seen as a secular analogy to the theological idea of *shalom*—a state of wholeness and well-being that transcends mere symptom relief. This shift from a focus on illness to health is potentially positive. However, this shift has a significant, if often unnoticed, problem.

Identifying some potential problems

There are hidden dangers in emphasizing mental health that should be noted. The movement away from using the language of mental *illness* as the sole way to describe mental health challenges is, in my view, helpful, especially considering how mental health diagnoses seem to be expanding, arguably turning general problems of living into mental illnesses, something we will return to later in this book. There is a real danger that *all of us* could end up defined as mentally ill. Nevertheless, the push for better mental health awareness brings with it some risks. The insidious nature of the mental health discourse is that while *some of us might be able to avoid the label of mental illness, none of us can escape the term "mental health."* But why, one might ask, would anyone *want* to escape that term? The idea of mental health seems benign. Why would we not want our lives to be defined by it?

The problem with mental health

Consider this perspective. It has likely not escaped the reader's notice that institutions such as universities, healthcare organizations, and businesses often implement mental health initiatives. These initiatives are typically accompanied by slogans like "*Your mental health matters*" and take the form of awareness weeks, mindfulness training, or stress-management workshops. On the surface, this may seem unproblematic, and in some ways it is not. However, despite the good intentions behind such initiatives, they possess a shadow side. If anxiety and depression are, at least in part, symptoms of the pressures created by these very institutions—by excessive workloads, unrealistic expectations, or exploitative practices—then the emphasis on *mental health* risks becoming a strategy of containment rather than transformation. Instead of addressing the root causes of distress, these initiatives merely help individuals adapt to a toxic environment. The system's response is not to question or reform the structures that produce psychological suffering, but to offer coping mechanisms that allow them to persist unchecked. In this way, the push toward *mental health* becomes less about genuine well-being and more about managing the symptoms of a deeper dysfunction—one that does not originate in individuals but emerges from unjust systems.

The contradiction is stark. On one hand, institutions promote the importance of mental health; on the other, they refuse to acknowledge that the real threat to well-being lies in their structures, policies, and economic priorities. The pressures of target-driven cultures, underfunded departments, the instrumentalization of staff and monetization of students create precisely the conditions that cause harm. Mindfulness, stress-reduction strategies, and resilience training may provide momentary relief, but they do nothing to challenge the systemic realities that necessitate these interventions in the first place.

The problem with resilience

Emphasizing mental health can easily foster a form of pathological resilience—one that, when viewed from a systemic perspective, tends to hinder rather than help. Resilience itself is not inherently harmful. However, when resilience is promoted as a means for individuals to adapt to unjust, economically driven, and hostile systems or poor working conditions, without addressing the systemic issues causing their struggles, it becomes oppressive. In such cases, mental health is no longer valued solely for enhancing individual well-being; instead, it transforms into an institutional expectation. Employees are implicitly *required* to maintain a state of mental health that aligns with the organization's demands.

Organizations may provide support to help individuals achieve a semblance of mental health, but this often translates to assisting them in adjusting to the system's pressures rather than addressing the root causes of distress. While the individuals leading these mental health initiatives may genuinely act with compassion, the broader institutional goal often prioritizes efficiency and productivity over genuine concern for personal well-being. If mental health were truly a priority, this would be reflected in the organization's overall structures and practices, not just in isolated mental health initiatives aimed at individuals.

The tension between the individual and the system

Having said this, it would be remiss of me not to acknowledge that counterforces exist to the individualization of mental health and ill health that I am highlighting here. While I argue that mainstream mental health discourse predominantly individualizes distress—emphasizing personal resilience, self-care, and individual coping strategies—I recognize that there is an increasing awareness of systemic and organizational factors that impact mental health. Various disciplines, including public health[1] and

[1] James B. Kirkbride, Diedre M. Anglin, Ian Colman, et al., "The Social Determinants of Mental Health and Disorder: Evidence, Prevention and Recommendations," *World Psychiatry* 23, no. 1 (2024): 58–90, doi:10.1002/wps.21160.

organizational psychology,[2] actively discuss how social structures, workplace cultures, and economic systems contribute to psychological distress and well-being.

Social determinants such as poverty, racial inequality, unstable housing, and adverse childhood experiences (ACEs) are crucial for understanding mental health and ill health. Similarly, organizational psychology increasingly investigates how toxic workplace cultures, job insecurity, and economic precarity create environments that worsen mental distress. Policy discussions within bodies such as the National Institute of Mental Health and the Substance Abuse and Mental Health Services Administration have aimed to move beyond purely individualized responses by incorporating systemic interventions such as trauma-informed care and workplace well-being policies.

[2] Melanie Genrich, Peter Angerer, Britta Worringer, et al., "Managers' Action-Guiding Mental Models Towards Mental Health-Related Organizational Interventions—A Systematic Review of Qualitative Studies," *International Journal of Environmental Research and Public Health* 19, no. 19 (2022): 12610, doi:10.3390/ijerph191912610.

The limits of systemic discourse in a neoliberal context

Nevertheless, although these systemic conversations exist, they often struggle against the prevailing framework of mental health discourse, which, as we shall see, is deeply embedded in neoliberal ideology. Speaking into the UK context, the psychiatrist Richard Bentall makes this point well in his book *Madness Explained.*[3] There he critiques the decline of social psychiatry, arguing that contemporary mental healthcare has largely abandoned its commitment to addressing the social causes of psychological distress. He notes that despite overwhelming evidence linking poverty, trauma, and inequality to conditions such as psychosis and depression, mainstream psychiatric practice remains dominated by biomedical and individualistic approaches. While research increasingly acknowledges that structural factors shape mental health, Bentall argues that such findings have rarely led to systemic interventions. Instead, they are typically used to refine individual-level treatments (such as cognitive-behavioral therapy [CBT] or medication) that focus on helping individuals cope with their circumstances rather

[3] Richard P. Bentall, *Madness Explained: Psychosis and Human Nature* (Allen Lane, 2003).

than transforming the conditions that generate distress. This reflects what Bentall sees as the narrowing of psychiatry's ambitions, where the field has shifted away from advocating for social change and has instead prioritized clinical strategies aimed at managing symptoms at the individual level. In doing so, mental health discourse risks becoming complicit in sustaining the very social inequalities that exacerbate psychological suffering rather than serving as a force for structural reform.

Thus, my argument is not that the language of mental health always ignores systemic factors, but that it tends to prioritize individual adaptation over collective transformation. Even in cases where systemic factors are acknowledged, solutions often emphasize personal coping strategies rather than substantive socioeconomic reform. This tension is at the heart of contemporary debates on mental healthcare: *Does it serve to liberate individuals from unjust systems, or does it function as a mechanism of social control, keeping individuals compliant within harmful structures?*

COULD WESTERN CULTURE BE BAD FOR OUR MENTAL HEALTH?

This question brings us to a broader and more provocative issue: *To what extent does Western culture itself contribute to the very mental distress it seeks to treat?* If, as I have argued, mainstream mental health discourse often prioritizes individual adaptation over systemic transformation, we must ask whether the dominant cultural and economic systems within which this discourse operates are themselves sources of psychological harm. Western societies, particularly those shaped by neoliberal ideology, celebrate personal responsibility, self-sufficiency, and resilience—values that, while not inherently negative, can become problematic when they obscure the reality that many forms of distress are socially produced. The emphasis on individual achievement and self-optimization, coupled with the erosion of communal structures and economic security, may exacerbate anxiety, loneliness, and depression rather than alleviating them. Moreover, the commodification of mental health—where well-being is marketed as a personal lifestyle choice requiring self-discipline, mindfulness apps, and wellness products—further reflects how deeply Western culture frames mental distress as a *personal failing* rather than a structural problem. In such a context, systemic solutions are not only neglected but actively resisted, as they challenge the ideological foundations of a culture built on competition and self-reliance. With this in mind, we must consider: *Is Western culture itself making us mentally unwell?* If so, how might we reimagine mental health in ways that resist its co-option into neoliberal individualism and instead foster genuine collective well-being?

The marketplace of the mind

The concerns I have raised about mental health stem from the reality that institutions such as healthcare services—once intended to prioritize the well-being of individuals for its own sake—have increasingly transformed into markets, operating similarly to industries like oil or steel. Within this economic paradigm, staff and patients, whether implicitly or explicitly, are treated as commodities, their value measured by their efficiency and productivity rather than by their intrinsic dignity and flourishing. In such a cultural landscape, mental health initiatives inevitably become individualized, centering on personal resilience and self-management rather than addressing the structural forces that generate distress. This observation will be crucial as we continue our exploration.

The contrast between this market-driven approach to mental health and the shalomic vision of human flourishing outlined in chapters 1 and 2 is striking. The former reduces well-being to an issue of individual optimization within an impersonal system, while the latter emphasizes the interdependent nature of human life—calling us to cultivate wholeness in relationship with God, community, and creation. One model seeks to help individuals survive within systems that prioritize efficiency over compassion, while the other envisions mental health as a shared, communal pursuit rooted in love and justice. The dissonance becomes even more profound when we examine these insights within the broader sociocultural landscape.

Mental health across cultures

It is well established that mental health challenges manifest differently across cultures.[4] Conditions such as depression, anorexia, posttraumatic stress disorder, and schizophrenia are not only diagnosed but also *experienced and treated* in ways deeply shaped by cultural context.[5] These discrepancies

[4] Arthur Kleinman, "Do Psychiatric Disorders Differ in Different Cultures?" In *Understanding and Applying Medical Anthropology*, ed. Peter J. Brown and Svea Closser, 3rd ed. (Routledge, 2016), 300–310.

[5] N. B. Paul, J. E. Maietta, and D. N. Allen, "Cultural Considerations for Schizophrenia Spectrum Disorders II: Assessment and Treatment," in *Handbook of Cultural Factors in Behavioral Health*, ed. L. T. Benuto, F. R. Gonzalez, and J. Singer (Springer Nature, 2020), https://doi.org/10.1007/978-3-030-32229-8_27; Neil Krishan Aggarwal,

invite a deeper exploration of the cultural factors that shape mental health outcomes.[6]

Cultural variations in mental health are not mere academic curiosities; they have profound practical consequences. For instance, research consistently shows that recovery rates for schizophrenia are higher in non-Western contexts, a finding that

---

"The Cross-Cultural Dimensions of Psychosis," *Psychiatric Times* 39, no. 11 (2022), https://www.psychiatrictimes.com/view/the-cross-cultural-dimensions-of-psychosis; Laurence J. Kirmayer, "Cultural Variations in the Clinical Presentation of Depression and Anxiety: Implications for Diagnosis and Treatment," *Journal of Clinical Psychiatry* 62, suppl. 13 (2001): 22–28; Sing Lee, "Reconsidering the Status of Anorexia Nervosa as a Western Culture-Bound Syndrome," *Social Science & Medicine* 42, no. 1 (1996): 21–34; Laura Jobson, Shamsul Haque, Siti Zainab Abdullah, et al., "Examining Cultural Differences in the Associations Between Appraisals and Emotion Regulation and Post-Traumatic Stress Disorder in Malaysian and Australian Trauma Survivors," *International Journal of Environmental Research and Public Health* 19, no. 3 (2022): 1163, doi: 10.3390/ijerph19031163.

[6] While we can't explore this in depth here, it is also worth noting Ethan Watters's warning that the United States (and indeed the West more generally) has a problematic tendency to "globalize the Western mind," that is, to export Western mental health frameworks and assume their universal applicability. This approach often imposes Western interpretations on cultures with their own nuanced understandings of mental health, effectively colonizing their ways of thinking.

challenges the assumption that Western psychiatric models are universally effective.[7] These discrepancies demand deeper exploration: What cultural factors enable greater recovery in certain societies? And why does the Western model often struggle to achieve similar outcomes despite its technological and medical advancements?

Thinking differently about symptoms: The symptom pool

To understand how and why symptoms and experiences differ across time and culture, it is helpful to turn to the work of historian Edward Shorter and his concept of *the symptom pool*. In his research on the history of anorexia, Shorter developed the metaphor of the symptom pool[8] to illustrate the various ways in which conditions are understood throughout

[7] Atalay Alem, Derege Kebede, Abebaw Fekadu, et al., "Clinical Course and Outcome of Schizophrenia in a Predominantly Treatment-Naive Cohort in Rural Ethiopia," *Schizophrenia Bulletin* 35 (2009): 646–54, doi:10.1093/schbul/sbn029. For a more critical account see Alex Cohen, Vikram Patel, R. Thara, and Oye Gureje, "Questioning an Axiom: Better Prognosis for Schizophrenia in the Developing World?" *Schizophrenia Bulletin* 34 (2008): 229–44, doi:10.1093/schbul/sbm105.

[8] Edward Shorter, "The First Great Increase in Anorexia Nervosa," *Journal of Social History* 21, no. 1 (1987): 69–96.

history. According to Shorter, the symptom pool comprises the set of symptoms that are culturally recognized and accepted at any given time. He argues that this symptom pool can change as cultural attitudes and medical understandings evolve. Shorter's thesis suggests that patients tend to present symptoms congruent with those acknowledged by the medical and cultural authorities of their time.

Every culture has a pool of symptoms available to its members. Members of that culture can choose—mainly through an unconscious process—which symptoms they will use to manifest their mental health experiences. Conditions rise and decline as people learn to pay attention to them in different ways or stop paying attention to them altogether. For instance, in the nineteenth century, female patients frequently exhibited symptoms like fainting and hysteria, which were common and accepted diagnoses at that time.[9] As the medical community's understanding changed and those diagnoses fell out of favor, the prevalence of such symptoms also decreased.

[9] Jon Stone, Russell Hewett, Alan Carson, Charles Warlow, and Michael Sharpe, "The 'Disappearance' of Hysteria: Historical Mystery or Illusion?" *Journal of the Royal Society of Medicine* (2008): 12–18, https://doi.org/10.1258/jrsm.2007.070129.

In his book *Mad Travellers*, philosopher Ian Hacking explored the brief appearance in the 1890s of a so-called *fugue state*, in which European men would walk in a trance for hundreds of miles, unaware of their identities.[10] These symptoms later disappeared, and the condition seems to no longer exist. Because these symptoms are unavailable, it has ceased to be an option for people or a potential diagnosis.

The anthropologist Arthur Kleinman conducted fieldwork and interviews in Taiwan during the 1970s, focusing on neurasthenia, a psychiatric diagnosis common in Chinese societies. He discovered that many Taiwanese people expressed emotional distress through physical symptoms rather than psychological ones. He argued that somatization (expressing distress through physical symptoms) served as a culturally shaped "idiom of distress" in Chinese culture. Kleinman found that individuals with depression in Taiwan often described their symptoms as problems with nerves, headaches, dizziness, pain, or weakness. They tended to seek care from traditional healers or physicians instead of psychiatrists. He suggested that somatization allowed

[10] Ian Hacking, *Mad Travellers: Reflections on the Reality of Transient Mental Illnesses*, new ed. (Harvard University Press, 2002).

Taiwanese individuals to convey distress in a manner that was more socially acceptable, thus avoiding the stigma associated with psychiatric conditions. Cultural attitudes towards mental health shaped the symptom pool available to Taiwanese people, where having a bodily condition was viewed as less stigmatizing than having a mental condition.

The French anthropologist Evelyne Pewzner-Apeloig found that the feeling of guilt, typically regarded as a core feature of depressive thinking, is less prevalent in cultures with a collective system of meaning than in individualistic societies.[11] Guilt can also manifest as a component of depression for theological reasons. Chaplain Iain McRitchie suggested that Calvinist doctrines of predestination, original sin, and an angry, wrathful God foster pessimism, guilt, and despair among believers. He claimed that the Calvinist perspective, which suggests that God predestines some for salvation and others for damnation, causes significant psychological distress as individuals continually question whether they are among the damned. Viewing the harsh and unforgiving nature of Calvinist teachings as contributing to

[11] Evelyne Pewzner-Apeloig, "The Occidental Model of Madness: A Critical Approach to the Concept of Ethnopsychiatry," *Annales Medico-Psychologique* (Paris) 151, no. 1 (1993): 64–74.

depression and hopelessness, McRitchie concluded that strong Calvinist religious beliefs and doctrines led to higher levels of depression and suicidal ideation in certain areas of the Scottish Highlands. He advocated for reforming Calvinism to be more positive and uplifting. The point here, in relation to our current conversation, is that guilt became a component of depression due to the prevalence of specific religious beliefs.[12]

Symptom adaptability

People tend to gravitate toward symptoms that are high on the scale of acceptable possibilities within any given culture. The historian of science Anne Harrington points out that such symptom adaptability is a necessary function for humans as cultural beings:

> Our bodies are physiologically primed to be able to do this, and for good reason: if we couldn't, we would risk not being taken seriously or not being cared for. Human beings seem to be invested with a developed capacity to mould their bodily

[12] I. A. M. Macritchie, "Celtic Culture, Calvinism, Social and Mental Health on the Island of Lewis," *Journal of Religion and Health* 33, no. 3 (1994): 269–78, http://www.jstor.org/stable/27510822.

> experiences to the norms of their cultures; they learn the scripts about what kinds of things should be happening to them as they fall ill and about the things they should do to feel better, and then they literally embody them.[13]

Recognizing this symptom adaptability helps us understand why mental health challenges manifest differently over time and across locations.

The power to create or disregard symptoms

This process of choosing symptoms and forming symptoms is not neutral. Those who seek to minister to the mentally unwell—be they doctors, chaplains, ministers, shamans, or anyone else—implicitly or explicitly encourage people to adopt specific symptoms and disregard others. Take myalgic encephalitis (ME)/Chronic Fatigue Syndrome (CFS) as a case in point. For many years, the medical profession did not accept those with ME symptoms—extreme tiredness, slow recovery after activity, and problems sleeping—as genuinely unwell. It took many years of fighting before this syndrome was accepted and recognized as officially existent. It only became "real" when the powerful voice of medicine began to take

[13] Anne Harrington, *The Cure Within: A History of Mind-Body Medicine* (W. W. Norton, 2008), 115.

it seriously, despite the fact that it had already been very real for those who suffered from it. Only when medicine officially recognized its existence was it possible to become an ME sufferer.[14]

An example of symptom formation and replacement within the realm of spirituality is ascribing demonic influences to the symptoms of mental health challenges such as psychosis. In this context, standard psychiatric explanations for a person's symptoms and experiences are dismissed and replaced by interpretations derived from religious traditions. Consequently, a new category of symptoms is introduced to the symptom pool: *the demonic*. Influential figures, such as pastors, ministers, or priests, attribute new meanings to these symptoms, overwhelming vulnerable individuals who may feel pressured

[14] Ian Hacking's concept of "making up people" highlights how classifications in the human sciences shape individual and collective experiences by creating new ways for people to understand themselves and be understood by society. The case of myalgic encephalomyelitis exemplifies this, as its classification legitimized patients' experiences and influenced policy, healthcare, and social attitudes. However, it also illustrates Hacking's warning about reductionism, where categories can constrain understanding and perpetuate stereotypes, particularly in contested illnesses. For more see Ian Hacking, "Making Up People," *London Review of Books* 28, no. 16 (2006): 23–26.

to adopt this new perspective—with potentially dangerous outcomes. As a result, medication may be rejected, and spiritual interventions such as exorcism become the presumed norm. The implications of this shift can be devastating. Expanding the symptom pool is not necessarily beneficial. Thus, the symptom pool is understood to be dynamic, expanding and contracting in response to both lay and professional interpretations and understandings.

New illnesses, new symptoms

Changes to the symptom pool are not always in response to new scientific developments. The pool sometimes changes as people change their opinions. The regular modifications in diagnostic criteria in the Diagnostic and Statistical Manual for Mental Disorders (DSM) are a good example of this. Homosexuality ceased to be classified as a mental illness in 1973 following pressure from gay-rights groups. In 1980 PTSD became a diagnosis following pressure from groups who worked to raise attention and support for those exposed to trauma.[15] Asperger's was removed from the DSM-5 by consensus, meaning it no longer officially exists. These changes are not the

[15] U.S. Department of Veteran Affairs, PTSD: National Center for PTSD, https://www.ptsd.va.gov/understand/what/history_ptsd.asp, last updated January 10, 2025.

result of new science but of the changing opinions of culture and psychiatry. The symptom pool is thus seen to expand or contract depending on how those with the power to name symptoms decide to frame people's experiences at any given moment.

We now begin to see how and why the kind of focus on mental health we discussed earlier places a certain interpretive slant on the symptom pool available to people working within organizations. It internalizes and individualizes causality and shapes the symptoms, making them a matter of personal welfare rather than corporate responsibility. When powerful organizations choose to name and define something like stress and anxiety in the workplace as symptoms of *individual* psychological malfunction, this places a particular interpretation on the cultural symptom pool, focusing attention on individual minds and diverting it away from corporate failures. It also enables, and perhaps even forces, people to adopt this way of naming their experiences, which may be part of the reason why stress and anxiety are so prevalent. People choose or are encouraged to label problems in their lives that are beyond their control as symptoms of personal pathology. The idea that their personal pathology may reflect a wider cultural pathology is rarely considered.

This discussion of the symptom pool helps us understand why mental health challenges vary across time and culture. Different cultures possess distinct theories of mind, unique symptom pools, and diverse responses to symptoms. It also highlights the culturally specific nature of Western approaches to mental health, which are shaped by particular views of the mind and methods for developing and addressing symptom pools. Despite the observation in chapter 2 that we are fundamentally corporate beings, Western mental health discourse often overemphasizes individual minds relative to collective symptoms or shared societal pathologies. The notion that broader cultural dynamics may contribute to mental health issues, as I have suggested, is present within the discourse but easily overshadowed by the dominant individualistic focus.

WHY NEOLIBERALISM AND CLIMATE CHANGE ARE BAD FOR OUR MENTAL HEALTH

Western cultures have significantly reshaped the symptom pool, reflecting the deep interconnection between mental health, the formation of symptoms, and prevailing political and economic ideologies. In particular, the ideology of neoliberal economics—emphasizing individualism, competition, commodification, and market-driven priorities—has profoundly influenced how mental health is understood and experienced, especially within Western societies, but increasingly so elsewhere due to the impact of globalization. This ideological framework shapes not only the symptoms people express but also the ways in which mental health challenges are addressed, often prioritizing individual solutions over systemic change. The sociologist of religion Matthew Guest, in his work on neoliberalism and religion, describes neoliberalism as referring to

> a set of cultural conditions indebted to the principles of neoliberal economics. These conditions may be summarized as a heightened individualism that prioritizes the freedom of the consumer over shared identities, a taken for granted assumption that market competition is the best measure of value and a tendency to treat cultural objects as commodities.[16]

Neoliberalism is not just an economic system; it is also an ideology and a worldview. A neoliberal worldview is characterized by increased individualism, where individuals define themselves in terms

[16] Mathew Guest, *Neoliberal Religion* (Bloomsbury, 2022), 7.

of freedom *from* others rather than freedom *for* others. It emphasizes *competition*, which pits one person against another in all aspects of life and society; *commodification*, the practice of transforming things into commodities that can be bought and sold; and *globalization*, which describes how technology has made the world deeply interconnected and interdependent. It is easy to understand how those within this system who are unable to meet its criteria will struggle to find sources of respect, value, and self-worth. Additionally, it's not difficult to recognize how the implicit anthropology of this system stands in stark contrast to the interpersonal, corporate model of personhood and flourishing we explored in chapters 1 and 2.

Mental health and neoliberalism

It is unsurprising, then, that there is a close connection between neoliberalism and the types of mental health vulnerabilities experienced by groups affected by its consequences. Race,[17] class,[18] and gender[19] have

[17] Anna Zeira, "Mental Health Challenges Related to Neoliberal Capitalism in the United States," *Community Mental Health Journal* (2022): 205–12, https://doi.org/10.1007/s10597-021-00840-7.

[18] Philip Browning Helsel, "Social Class and Mental Illness in a Neoliberal Era," in *Pastoral Power Beyond Psychology's Marginalization: Resisting the Discourses of the Psy-Complex* (Springer, 2015), 19–51.

[19] Julia Coffey, "Ugly Feelings: Gender, Neoliberalism and the Affective Relations of Body Concerns," *Journal*

all been negatively impacted by neoliberal economics and its accompanying worldview. If economic success is taken as the principal measure of human worth and the good life, then failure to achieve such success is construed not merely as misfortune but as a fundamental deficiency in being—a failure of life itself. Worse still, if one fails due to the inherent push against collectivism and the reduction of government intervention, the necessary safety nets may not be present. Even more troubling, *others will blame those who do not appear economically successful for their situation.*[20] Since mental ill-health is seen as a *personal* weakness impacting individual minds, people will find themselves without support and no

---

of Gender Studies 29, no. 6 (2020): 636–50.

[20] Dana L. Cloud argues that therapeutic discourse shifts social and political problems into the realm of individual psychological adjustment, thereby discouraging collective action and systemic change. She critiques how the "rhetoric of therapy" promotes personal coping mechanisms instead of addressing the structural conditions that generate suffering. By encouraging individuals to seek self-improvement rather than societal transformation, therapy-oriented rhetoric reinforces neoliberal ideologies that prioritize personal responsibility over collective justice. This process ultimately depoliticizes social struggle, making systemic inequalities seem like personal burdens rather than issues requiring political and structural solutions. Dana L. Cloud, *Control and Consolation in American Culture and Politics: Rhetoric of Therapy* (Sage, 1998).

one to blame but themselves. In such a system, corporate pathogens manifest in individual minds.

New forms of "old" conditions

Unsurprisingly, this economic system and its accompanying practices are reshaping and expanding the symptom pool. In his book *Caring for Souls in a Neoliberal Age*, Bruce Rogers-Vaughn offers an important critique of neoliberalism as it relates to pastoral care,[21] pointing out that neoliberalism is altering the nature of suffering. He provides a framework for understanding suffering that differentiates three distinct types: first, second, and third-order suffering.

First-order suffering

First-order suffering refers to the suffering that results directly from specific events or conditions. This encompasses physical pain, emotional distress, and psychological anguish stemming from experiences such as illness, loss of a loved one, natural disasters, and violence. First-order suffering is often immediate and can typically be observed directly.

Second-order suffering

Second-order suffering is not caused directly by events or conditions; instead, it arises from how

[21] Bruce Rogers-Vaughn, *Caring for Souls in a Neoliberal Age* (Palgrave Macmillan, 2016), ch. 4.

we interpret or ascribe meaning to first-order suffering—the personal and existential interpretations we associate with pain and adversity. For instance, if someone perceives their suffering as punishment or as a sign of a meaningless universe, that layer of interpretation introduces a second order of suffering.

Third-order suffering

Third-order suffering represents a new form of suffering—a collective or systemic type that emerges from the societal structures and cultural narratives shaping our lives. It encompasses systemic injustices, social sins, and institutional forms of violence that inflict pain on individuals and groups. This type of suffering is often less visible compared to others at an individual level, yet it is pervasive and can profoundly impact large groups of people, often in insidious ways. Recognizing and addressing third-order suffering can be challenging, but understanding its role in perpetuating cycles of suffering is crucial.

Neoliberal ideology, Rogers-Vaughn suggests, contributes significantly to third-order suffering. By reducing and fragmenting human subjects, stripping them of their collectivist impulses, and starving them of the kind of narratives that helped people make sense of suffering in previous generations, it shapes suffering in very specific ways. According to Rogers-Vaughn,

> Without strong, vibrant collectives to support them, individuals are more-or-less left to their own devices to deal with distress. We might describe them as in a state of *spiritual homelessness*. These unfortunate souls are abandoned, left to interpret their sufferings as signs of personal failure. They are not guilty. They are ashamed. They do not have adequate narrative resources at hand to understand, to "make sense of," their sufferings. They are left simply with market-generated narratives of "personal recovery" . . . which, like insulin for the diabetic, are perpetually fragile in the face of what they are up against. Such narratives are window-dressing, a veneer of order imposed over what once would have been a durable sense of self. The terms used to describe first- and second-order suffering now fail them, largely because the sources of their sufferings are no longer easily identified. Their oppressors, for example, no longer have faces, even the impersonal "faces" of the state, the corporation, or the church. Yet to say

> the oppressor is some abstract "evil" seems not to capture the thing.[22]

People suffer in a strange, anomic, narrative-starved state that, some have noted, is a significant driver not only for anxiety and depression but also for suicide.[23]

Importantly, third-order suffering changes the symptom pool by altering the shape of first- and second-order suffering. Depression is becoming more diffuse and unfocused. Anxiety is becoming more and more amorphous. Addictions are more fluid and vaguer. The answers to big questions—Who am I? Where do I come from? Where am I going? Why?—now tend to be defined in relation to the presence or absence of personal success . . . which is largely determined by fluctuations of the market. Even when a person is doing well, they may suffer from new forms of anxiety such as "recession anxiety,"[24] a form of anxiety that comes from being at the mercy of the markets and knowing that everything one has

[22] Rogers-Vaughn, *Caring for Souls*, 126.

[23] Anne Case and Angus Deaton, *Deaths of Despair and the Future of Capitalism* (Princeton University Press, 2021).

[24] Pam Belluck, "Recession Anxiety Seeps into Everyday Lives," *New York Times*, April 9, 2009, https://www.nytimes.com/2009/04/09/health/09stress.html.

they could lose if the economy goes bust. People are experiencing a diffuse and fragmented self, defined not by any form of real-life community or collectivist activity but *by themselves.*

But even self-definition has become complicated. With the rise of social media and the constant push to gauge one's success based on how others perceive you—red hearts and thumbs up/likes on your social media page—your sense of self is perpetually at risk in the marketplace of external observers who may buy into your presented self-image, yet who could also cancel you at a moment's notice. This leads to overwhelming anxiety and depression, the sources of which are not always identifiable, which in turn heightens our anxiety. *Why am I anxious!?* In such situations, it is easy to start assuming that if the source of my failure is not external, it must be internal. *I* am the problem. Despite the fact that the issue may (as we have seen) lie within the structures of wider society, shame in the face of personal failure is a burden that many find challenging to bear. And of course, for the reasons outlined earlier, our mental healthcare responses tend to focus on helping individuals and healing individual minds rather than changing culture, thus risking the reinforcement of this sense of the intrapersonal locus of pathology.

Creating the conditions for the internalization of social problems, building a model of personhood that depends on winning at all costs, and failing to provide a meaningful narrative to explain people's anomie, anxiety, fear, and depression are all significant ways in which neoliberalism has been reshaping the symptom pool. It's not that conditions like anxiety and depression are new; rather, within a neoliberal context, they assume a new shape and form, necessitating different, more corporate and systems-wide responses and interventions alongside standard personal approaches. Exploring what this might entail will be the focus of the final chapter of this book.

Creating new conditions

Yet there is more. It is not only that symptoms are being revised and reconfigured within a neoliberal worldview; new conditions are coming into existence. Chapters 1 and 2 demonstrated that we are designed to live in harmony/shalom with one another and with creation. To live in shalom is to care well for one another and to take care of creation. Disruption in our relationship with creation will lead to disruption in other areas of our lives. One consequence of a neoliberal worldview is that the sacredness of creation fades as the land, seas, and skies (even space!) are viewed as commodities to be bought, sold, exploited, and controlled. The commodification of creation has resulted in the degradation of ecosystems across the globe, the depletion of natural resources such as water, air, and soil, the destruction of rainforests, the acidification of our seas, the mass extinction of species, and unprecedented floods, hurricanes, fires, and other disastrous events caused by changes in our climate.

Ecoanxiety

The destruction of the land, seas, and skies has a profound and negative impact on mental health, disrupting the sense of harmony and shalomic interconnectedness essential to human well-being. This relationship is well documented in reports by the American Psychological Association, which highlight how ecological degradation contributes to conditions such as ecoanxiety, climate-related stress, and other mental health challenges.[25] This ecological destruction has brought with it new configurations of symptoms and the formation of new conditions. For example, we now talk about *ecoanxiety* or *climate*

[25] At the time of this writing, the most recent report is "Addressing the Climate Crisis: An Action Plan for Psychologists," Report of the APA Task Force on Climate Change (2022), https://www.apa.org/science/about/publications/climate-crisis-action-plan.pdf.

anxiety.[26] Ecoanxiety is a redirection of previous understandings of anxiety and a significant reconfiguration of the symptom pool. A sense of panic marks this form of anxiety, worry, and fear about the consequences of ecological damage. Ecoanxiety and climate anxiety are not exactly the same, for to be anxious about the ecological state of the world does not necessitate the acceptance of the theory of climate change, but they are interconnected. Both are shaped by our environment, by the media, social media, and other sources of knowledge. Both are particularly strong among young people. Due to the rise of social media and 24/7 news, we do not have to be directly involved with ecological damage for it to affect our mental health; we merely have to be aware of it.

Homelessness at home

The commodification and damaging of creation have also *contributed* to the symptom pool. An example of this is *solastalgia*, an idea advanced by Australian

[26] Amidon Lusted Marcia, *Coping with Ecoanxiety* (Rosen, 2021), https://public.ebookcentral.proquest.com/choice/publicfullrecord.aspx?p=5971535; see also Britt Wray and Adam McKay, *Generation Dread: Finding Purpose in an Age of Climate Anxiety* (Experiment, 2023), https://public.ebookcentral.proquest.com/choice/PublicFullRecord.aspx?p=30552278.

environmental philosopher Glenn Albrecht in response to ecological destruction and radical changes in the Australian environment. His original focus was on the experiences of Indigenous Australians and rural farmers, both of whom were facing profound ecological change and the intentional destruction of their land for profit. As the ecosystem in which these people lived and worked came under stress, they began to experience significant psychological and existential distress, or what eco-philosopher Edward S. Casey has described as "place pathology"—a form of existential lostness that comes when one loses one's sense of place. Casey had displaced people in mind, but Albrecht noticed this kind of place pathology was also present in people who were still at home, in the same place, but who could no longer recognize or feel connected to that place. The symptoms of this place pathology included a particular form of anxiety, depression, hopelessness, and existential emptiness. They were at home in their land, but their land no longer felt like home.

The term *solastalgia* contains a ghost reference to nostalgia (*nostos* = return home; *algia* = pain or sickness). The term *nostalgia* used to be linked to the diagnosis of melancholia as it related to people's homesickness when distant from home:[27]

[27] Glenn Albrecht, "'Solastalgia': A New Concept in Health and Identity," *PAN: Philosophy, Activism, Nature* 3 (2005): 41–55 (45).

> Nostalgia . . . or literally, the sickness caused by the inability to return home, was considered to be a medically diagnosable psycho-physiological disease right up to the middle of the C20. In 1905 nostalgia was defined as: . . . a feeling of melancholy caused by grief on account of absence from one's home country, of which the English equivalent is homesickness.[28]

Nostalgia is particularly strong in people who have been forced to leave their land. For example, soldiers who are compelled to fight in foreign lands can be completely incapacitated by homesickness, as can refugees displaced by war, immigrants, or individuals affected by climate change, violence, or economic hardships. However, nostalgia isn't merely a longing for lost times; it is also a yearning for lost places. This is especially relevant for Indigenous communities whose lands have been destroyed and whose history has been rendered insignificant. The same sentiment applies to anyone who feels dispossessed of their homeland, even if they are still physically at home.

Albrecht combined the notions of nostalgia (a longing for home), solace (the alleviation of distress), and desolation (abandonment and loneliness) to define solastalgia as "the pain or sickness caused

[28] Albrecht, "Solastalgia," 42.

by the loss or lack of solace and the sense of isolation connected to the present state of one's home and territory." As noted, this term was originally applied to the ecological experiences of Indigenous Australians and rural farmers facing environmental destruction. However, solastalgia extends to a wide range of situations in which an individual's sense of place and identity is undermined. This distress is often most acute when people directly witness the devastation of their environment. Nonetheless, even indirect exposure—through media coverage of fires, floods, wars, or pollution—can evoke a profound sense of loss and displacement. In this way, solastalgia transcends individual experiences, becoming a collective phenomenon that highlights how ecological destruction, social upheaval, and cultural change disrupt the deep connections between place, identity, and mental health. The concept offers a vital framework for recognizing and addressing the psychological impacts of living in a world that feels increasingly fragile and unfamiliar.

The interplay between this psychological phenomenon and political ideologies such as neoliberalism reveals the complex ways in which perceptions of "home" and belonging are tied not just to physical geography but to cultural and social identity. In this sense, solastalgia extends beyond individual experiences of ecological loss to encompass collective responses to broader societal transformations, highlighting the deeply intertwined nature of place, identity, and mental health. This way of thinking about nostalgia also resonates in interesting ways with Rogers-Vaughn's thinking about the anomie of neoliberal culture.

Solastalgia is an extremely complex phenomenon that affects not only those who have lost their homeland but also those who perceive their country or community as undergoing rapid and unsettling change. Albrecht's concept of solastalgia offers a lens to understand this broader experience of existential displacement. For many, distress stems not from physical dislocation but from a profound sense that their once-familiar environment—whether ecological, cultural, or societal—is becoming unrecognizable.

This sense of alienation is evident in contemporary political movements, particularly the rightward shift in Europe in response to a historic rise in immigration. As communities grapple with significant demographic and economic changes, some individuals experience a form of collective solastalgia marked by anxiety and fear over the perceived erosion of familiar norms and traditions. These reactions underscore how the destabilization of one's sense of place—be it through environmental degradation or societal transformation—can trigger psychological distress with profound personal and political consequences.

CONCLUSION

A holistic approach to mental healthcare, grounded in the rich and expansive vision of shalom, demands that we move beyond a narrow focus on individual challenges and symptoms. It requires us to address the interwoven social, political, economic, and ecological realities shaping our mental health and well-being. This chapter has demonstrated that systemic injustice, cultural instability, and ecological destruction are not peripheral concerns but central factors in the formation of mental distress. Recognizing these broader dynamics compels us to reimagine mental healthcare as a communal and systemic endeavor rather than a solely individualized pursuit.

To truly care for people's mental health faithfully, we must go deeper: addressing the root causes of suffering and fostering environments where individuals and communities can flourish. A shalomic vision calls us to seek justice in the structures that shape our world, cultivate belonging in fractured communities, and restore harmony with creation. This multidimensional approach is not merely an ideal—it is an ethical imperative for those who wish to bring meaningful healing and hope into a broken world.

In the final chapter we will move from theory to practice, exploring actionable strategies for embodying this holistic vision. Drawing on insights from pastoral care and theology, we will consider how faith communities, caregivers, and institutions can create spaces where healing is not just about symptom relief but about restoring relationships—with God, with others, and with creation. The journey toward shalom is complex but also deeply transformative.

4
FINDING PEACE WITH GOD

A Deeper, Kinder Theology of Mental Health

When viewed through the lens of shalom, we recognize mental health and mental healthcare as complex and diverse, with far-reaching implications for individuals, communities, and creation. Caring for individuals remains crucial, as do our current methods of helping people find healing, even if our ideas of what an individual is changes as we reflect on the harmonious interconnection of shalomic flourishing. Individuals matter but taking care of the places where individuals live their lives and recognizing the importance of these places as loci for the formation of mental health and ill-health is equally important. In this final chapter I begin to explore the implications of such findings for the practices of Christians who seek to engage in faithful mental healthcare and embody the vision of shalom-as-mental health. I'm not suggesting that we all become outspoken critics of capitalism or devoted environmental activists—unless, of course, that is your calling. It is unlikely (but not impossible) that you or I will change the powerful systems of this world which cause so much pain, injustice, and suffering. Ultimately, that is God's job. We—the body of Jesus—must do everything we can, but we can't do everything. Thomas Merton once wrote: "Our job is to love others without stopping to inquire whether or not they are worthy."[1] There is great power in these words. As creatures made by love, for love, and rooted and grounded in love (Eph 3:17), our calling is to participate in the loving, shalomic mission of Jesus in, to, and for the world—a mission that changes things not by might, nor by power, but by the Spirit of God (Zech 4:1). Such love may appear foolish in the face of the enormity of the troubles of this world. And yet, small gestures can reveal powerful things (Matt 17:20). When we center our thinking on love—for ourselves, our neighbor, creation, and God—the practices of faithful mental healthcare emerge in new and transformative ways. In what

[1] Thomas Merton, *Disputed Questions* (Harcourt Brace Jovanovich, 1985).

follows, I will suggest four areas for our consideration in response to the arguments laid out in the earlier parts of this book, namely that we:

(1) learn to live kindly and think corporately;

(2) decommodify our minds;

(3) strive to bring healing to the symptom pool in order that people can live healthily even amidst suffering and distress; and

(4) love our neighbor and our future neighbors.

While these four things are clearly not a comprehensive strategy, they can launch a deeper, kinder, and more practical theology of mental health. Every journey begins with a first step.

LIVING KINDLY, THINKING CORPORATELY

In chapters 1 and 2 we explored the importance of recognizing human beings as relational creatures, deeply embedded in community and dependent on the presence of others. We live our lives together. We share our minds together. Here, I want to suggest that central to the peace-bringing dynamic of shalom is a particular way of being with one another that reflects and communicates its intricate mutuality: *the way of kindness.*

Kindness is an essential dynamic of shalom. It is both a gift of the Spirit and a way of being in the world that shapes us into the image of Jesus. Paul urges us in Ephesians 4:31–32: "*Put away from you all bitterness and wrath and anger and wrangling and slander, together with all malice. Be kind to one another, tenderhearted, forgiving one another, as God in Christ has forgiven you*" (NRSV). Kindness reflects the character of God, revealed most fully in Jesus Christ. As Titus 3:4–5 reminds us: "*But when the goodness and loving kindness of God our Savior appeared, he saved us, not because of any works of righteousness that we had done, but according to his mercy*" (NRSV). This divine kindness, expressed in Christ's saving work, calls us to embody the same grace and love in our lives.

Kindness is also a fruit of the Spirit, as Galatians 5:22–23 states: "*The fruit of the Spirit is love, joy, peace, patience, kindness, generosity, faithfulness, gentleness, and self-control*" (NRSV). Clothed in kindness, as Colossians 3:12 instructs, we live out our vocation as those made in the image of God. Spirit-filled kindness is no mere sentiment; it is a powerful, transformative force that can reshape relationships, communities, and even systems. It is the overflow of God's love within us, enabling acts of grace, forgiveness, and compassion that transcend human limitations. Kindness has the power to heal wounds, bridge divides, and restore dignity. It is a profound reflection of God's presence, working through us to bring about the harmony of shalom. Kindness reminds us of who we are and *whose* we are. It anchors us in the love of God and empowers us to extend that love to others. In doing so, it fosters healing, connection, and the flourishing of community, revealing the very heart of God in our shared lives.

Kindness reminds us of who we are and whose we are.

The problem of unkindness

I use the term "kindness" here in two interconnected ways. The first relates to kindness as a practice—something that God's creatures *do*. When we reflect on the issues we have explored earlier, we can see that at their heart is a fundamental lack of kindness towards self, others, and all of creation. The reason many people experience mental health problems is because their lives have been the subject of much *un*kindness, either during their early years or at some other point in their life's journey. The problems they hold within their bodies are testimony to the unkindness of others.[2] The lone-

[2] This aligns with the arguments around trauma in Bessel A. Van der Kolk, *The Body Keeps the Score: Brain, Mind, and Body in the Healing of Trauma* (Penguin Books, 2014).

liness and isolation that many people with mental health challenges experience emerge from the ways in which society constructs mental health challenges in deeply negative and unkind ways.[3] These constructions are not intrinsic to a person's condition; rather, they are challenges that arise from the context in which the condition is experienced. The over-individualization of mental health challenges and the imposition of stigma based on a presumed difference between "them" and "us" is frankly and simply unkind as well as inappropriate and unnecessary. Assuming the personal without recognizing the corporate and systemic dimensions of mental health challenges allows broader society to abrogate responsibility, which in turn leads to distancing, shame, and unkindness.

The worldview and anthropology that emerge from the type of neoliberal politics and economics we explored in the previous chapter are deeply unkind, particularly toward the poorest and most vulnerable within our society. At the same time, they are *very* kind to those who benefit from the system and whose lives are often marked by extreme excess. This unkind system reveals itself in individuals being

[3] Ami Rokach, "Loneliness of the Marginalized," *Open Journal of Depression* 3 (2014): 147–53, doi:10.4236/ojd.2014.34018.

unkind to themselves, assuming that their problems are entirely down to them, something that, as we have seen, can be reinforced by certain ways of thinking about mental health. This leads to forms of shame and self-alienation, which layer themselves on top of already troubled individuals. Organizations, political systems, and economies that refuse to look downwards will always fail to be kind to those who are trapped below its gaze.

The anthropology that emerges from such systems is likewise unkind. The idea that we look toward ourselves and away from others, the presumption that others are foes and competitors rather than potential friends and fellow travelers, and the assumption that those who cannot achieve are wasting resources is an unkind way to frame human beings. The idea that our health and well-being can be framed in terms of lucrative markets rather than mutual moral responsibility results in systems and practices rampant with unkindness. And as we have seen, we are showing little kindness toward creation, with all the implications that such unkindness brings for our mental health. All these dimensions of unkindness cause profound disruption to God's shalom and fail to manifest the love, mercy, and kindness of Jesus toward the whole of the created order.

In chapter 2 I argued that minds are not self-contained units but rather relationally constructed realities. This means that unkindness—whether expressed through social exclusion, systemic injustice, or everyday interpersonal neglect—does not merely wound metaphorically; it actively reshapes neural pathways and alters the way people experience the world. A culture that tolerates or even normalizes unkindness is not just ethically flawed—it is neurobiologically and theologically destructive. It transforms our minds in negative ways. If minds emerge within relationships, then mental health cannot be an isolated pursuit but must be viewed as a shared moral responsibility marked by kindness. Practicing kindness in this context is a profound form of healing that counters such unkindness. The mental well-being of one is always interwoven with the mental well-being of the many.

The shape of kindness

Kindness is not only a compassionate action; it is also a statement about the nature of God and, by implication, the nature of human beings. The fourteenth-century English mystic and anchoress Julian of Norwich reminds us that: "*God is kind in his being: that is to say, that goodness that is kind, it is God . . . He is the same thing that is kindness, and he is the Father and Mother of kinds*."[4] Goodness is the kind of "thing" that God is. This is an important observation. The term *kindness*, as Julian uses it here, comes from Middle English in which the word has a complex set of meanings we rarely consider now:

> It indicates the benevolence that we mean today when we speak of someone as "kind"; it also indicates the nature of a thing, what "kind" of thing it is, as when we speak of "humankind"; and somewhere between benevolence and nature, it indicates the relationship between those who share a common nature—thus the words "kin" and "kindred." In any particular instance, the word "kind" may well carry all of these meanings. To say that someone treated you "kindly" would be to say that she acted in a benevolent way (kindly), as if you were her relative (kindred), and in a way that is only natural to someone like her (her kind). Julian's use of this term encompasses all of these meanings.[5]

[4] Julian of Norwich, *Revelations of Divine Love*, with a foreword by Kaya Oakes (Ixia Press, 2019), ch. 62.

[5] F. C. Bauerschmidt, "Order, Freedom, and 'Kindness': Julian of Norwich on the Edge of Modernity," *Theology Today* (2003): 63–81 (73).

Kindness is not simply something God *does*; it is something God *is*. *God is kind*. More than that, in Jesus's incarnation, God became our kind. As we come to know Jesus's kindness and understand Jesus as kin, we discover the sort of creatures we are.

In Jesus, we discover we are kin to one another, called to act kindly in a world created by a God who is kind. Kindness is thus more than simply compassionate action (although it is, of course, that): it is also the recognition of the *kind* of creatures we are, the kinship that we share with others and the kinship we share with creation as Jesus, in his kindness, seeks to bring about the redemption of all things (Col 1:20). As creatures made in the image of a kind God who in Jesus became our kind, kindness in all of its dimensions is part of the kind of thing we are.[6]

[6] The New Testament conveys kinship and kindness through distinct but interconnected themes. While Julian of Norwich draws on Middle English etymology, the New Testament expresses kinship through familial language, particularly in references to believers as "brothers and sisters" and "children of God" (Rom 8:15–17; Gal 4:5–7). Kindness is similarly emphasized as a fruit of the Spirit (Gal 5:22) and a moral imperative (Eph 4:32), reflecting God's benevolence. Hebrews 2:11 ties these themes together in Christ's incarnation, declaring that Jesus is not ashamed to call humanity his kin. Thus, while the NT does not explicitly use the terms "kindness" and "kinship" together, it affirms their theological unity: kindness is both an ethical imperative and a

Within the context of mental healthcare, acting kindly is the first step away from stigma and toward belonging. No matter how different people's experiences may be as they journey through their mental health challenges, people are always our kind and should always be treated kindly. There is no room for distancing and othering in a community of kindness. Kindness leads to the creation of communities where people *belong*, where their bodies are seen as bridges rather than barriers. People will certainly need professional help, and that should be welcomed. However, the role of the body of Christ is not primarily to deliver therapy. The task of the body of Jesus is to be kind and to remind people of their kind-ness.

THE BODY OF CHRIST HAS MENTAL HEALTH CHALLENGES

We can now begin to see why kindness sits at the very heart of shalom as mental health. When we recognize what kind of creatures we are—people who long to relate, belong, and be with others who act kindly—we can begin to act kindly toward one another. Likewise, when we realize what kind of minds we have, it pushes us to recognize the centrality of relationships for care of mind. Kindness

---

reflection of our shared identity as those made in the image of a kind God who, through Christ, became our kin.

encourages us to think *corporately*. The term *corporate* is used extensively in business and relates to large companies. It is very much tied to the neoliberal economic worldview we examined in the previous chapter. There is, however, another way in which we can think of the term "corporate": *acting together as a group rather than as separate individuals*. To act corporately is to act as one body. Recognizing the kind of people we are—namely, inherently relational stewards of creation—enables us to think and act corporately. To think corporately is to think with the mind of Christ. The ideas of the body of Christ and the mind of Christ we explored earlier draw our attention to the corporate nature of the Christian life. We are who we are in Christ, and we live into our kindness as we encounter the kindness of others. We suffer together, and we find healing together.

In contrast to the individualism and individualization of mental health challenges that seem to have become a norm for Westerners, thinking corporately about mental health issues allows those challenges to become shared experiences. Rather than only thinking in terms of individuals with mental health challenges (invaluable as individuals undoubtedly are), the community of kindness shares in the sufferings of the body. If one member of the body experiences a mental health challenge, we all do. In a real sense, *the body of Jesus has mental health challenges*. Thinking this way helps us avoid abandoning one another in times of need. When someone becomes unwell, our responsibility is not merely to acknowledge their suffering but to respond actively: to be present, to extend kindness, to visit with constancy, to seek genuine understanding, to assist in securing appropriate forms of care, and to offer the sustaining gift of friendship. Recognizing the shared ownership of mental health challenges also helps us avoid abandoning caregivers. Caring can be a very lonely and exhausting calling. If the body of Christ has mental health challenges, then the task of caring belongs to us all. The kindness of respite, accompaniment, friendship, and prayer all offer relief for people when the exhausting process of caring for someone who is languishing takes its toll. Kindness and corporate thinking lead to solidarity: *standing firm with one another*.

Finding sanctuary

In order to show solidarity and stand firm with one another, we, the church, must become a place of *sanctuary* and a place of prophetic action. Sanctuary refers to a refuge or safety from pursuit, persecution, or other danger. In a pathogenic and often actively hostile culture, sanctuary can be hard to find for people living with mental health challenges. As shalomic people driven by the kindness of God, *our calling as Christians is to become a sanctuary*. We need to become people who recognize cultural pathologies and wrestle through prayer, practice, and presence to provide safe places of sanctuary where those of us struggling with our mental health can encounter the kindness of shalom. Showing such solidarity and offering sanctuary does not mean annexation. People remain individuals able to make their own choices and live separate lives. It does, however, mean recognition of the interconnectedness of our minds and bodies and an intentional effort to live that out within the shalomic sanctuary of kindness.

Sanctuary does not mean escape from the world. In recognition of the kinds of issues I have highlighted in this book, it means responding to the call to offer a prophetic response and critique. I am not suggesting we all become political activists, although we should all always be engaged in the struggle to develop newer and fairer systems. I am, however, suggesting that we allow the Spirit to transform our minds in ways that enable us to function kindly in the midst of what is, as we have seen, a deeply challenging cultural worldview. An essential step toward such a goal is to learn to *decommodify our minds*.

Decommodifying our minds

In the previous chapter I noted the power of markets to commodify the world and to teach us how to understand worth, value, normality, and acceptable life direction. Briefly:

> Commodification describes the process by which something without an economic value gains economic value that can replace other social values. The process changes relationships that were previously untainted by commerce into relationships that essentially become commercial in everyday use.[7]

To commodify something or someone is to turn them into a unit whose value is gauged in terms of financial return. Commodification is an economic process, but it is also a way of looking at things and people—a mindset and a worldview.

While markets may rule our economic systems, they do not have to rule our minds. If we are to engage effectively in our mission of shalomic kindness, those of us who seek to share in the mind of Christ need

[7] Roger Levesque, "Commodification," in *Encyclopedia of Adolescence*, ed. Roger Levesque (Springer, 2018), https://doi.org/10.1007/978-3-319-32132-5_790-1.

to learn to decommodify our minds. Decommodification is the process of returning the original value to something or someone. It relates to reevaluating a commodity according to a different set of criteria not determined by market desires. Decommodification refers to forms of critical thinking that recognize and intentionally resist the commodifying tendencies of our systems. A decommodified mind strives to think with the mind of Christ, that is, to develop a mindset determined by kindness rather than by the values of the market. Decommodification does not mean withdrawing from the system of neoliberalism. It does, however, mean finding ways of resisting the anthropology and worldview this system creates and intentionally pushing against those aspects that are damaging to our mental health. Decommodification is a way of looking at the world which we should strive to implement in every aspect of our lives. It is something particularly important in relation to our highly commodified healthcare systems within which everything and everyone has become a commodity.

Decommodifying mental healthcare: The example of psychopharmacology

Modern mental healthcare is big business. Its structure comprises a variety of different markets within which people and things are commodified in ways intended to maximize financial gain and bring about acceptable mental health outcomes. The skills of clinicians are packaged, bought, and sold, as are the technologies they purchase and use. Time, effort, presence, and outcomes are all commodified, shaped and formed by the needs of internal and external markets. This comes with obvious tensions and temptations. If personal financial payments become marketing tools, the potential for implicit or explicit bias is obvious.[8] If we take as an example the pharmaceutical market, some of the issues around the importance of decommodified thinking will become clear.

The marketing of psychiatric medication is immensely lucrative. With that comes certain temptations. As new conditions enter the symptom pool through the DSM via the creation of lay diagnoses such as ecoanxiety and solastalgia or by people

[8] Ramin Mojtabai and Mark Olfson, "Proportion of Antidepressants Prescribed Without a Psychiatric Diagnosis Is Growing," *Health Affairs* 30, no. 8 (2011): 1434–42, doi: 10.1377/hlthaff.2010.1024; Marcia Angell, "Drug Companies and Doctors: A Story of Corruption," *New York Review of Books* 56, no. 1 (2009): 8–12; Thomas R. Insel, "Psychiatrists' Relationships with Pharmaceutical Companies: Part of the Problem or Part of the Solution?" *JAMA* 303, no. 12 (2010): 1192–93, doi:10.1001/jama.2010.317.

self-diagnosing via the internet, those conditions are soon accompanied by new medications or the rerouting or reappropriation of longstanding medications. As the push toward biological explanations of mental health challenges continues, so the temptation to develop codependent relationships between drug companies and biological psychiatry becomes alluring.[9] With the permitting of straight-to-customer selling of psychopharmacological products comes the temptation to move people away from evidence-based justifications for the giving or not giving of medication toward an emphasis on good marketing strategies based on the assumption that things like the presence of happiness and freedom from anxiety define the good life. To decommodify our thinking within this area, we must think corporately and kindly about what medication *is* and what it intends to *do*.

To be clear, *decommodifying medication does not mean ceasing to recommend or use medication and it certainly does not mean that we stop taking medication*. Medication is vital for many people. At the same time, the reasons for giving and receiving medication and its impact on people are also very important.

[9] John Read, "Schizophrenia, Drug Companies, and the Internet," *Social Science & Medicine* 66, no. 1 (2008): 99–109, 10.1016/j.socscimed.2007.07.027.

Our reflections in chapter 2 on Paul's perspective on body and mind revealed the centrality of the body as the ground of our personhood and how the body is foundationally relational and participatory. If that is so, the proper goal of psychopharmacology is not simply to deal with individual symptoms or behaviors that appear problematic for individuals or others (although it may, of course, involve this). The theological goal of psychopharmacology is to remove any barriers that prevent someone from engaging in the kinds of relationships and human connections that keep us healthy in our shared mind and corporate personhood. Medication, faithfully prescribed and administered, allows the development of what Susan Eastman describes as "life giving connection rather than self-directed, self-sufficient individualism."[10] If the motivation for giving and receiving medication has a particular theological goal, then alongside the standard clinical questions we ask when prescribing we should also consider asking another set of questions.

[10] Susan G. Eastman, "Bodies, Agency, and the Relational Self: A Pauline Approach to the Goals and Use of Psychiatric Drugs," *Christian Bioethics: Non-Ecumenical Studies in Medical Morality* 24, no. 3 (2018): 291, doi:10.1093/CB/CBY011.

Decommodifying prescribing

If we are to decommodify the practice of prescribing, prescribers should not simply ask: "Is this the cheapest drug that will control this particular feeling or behavior?" For this is a question that focuses on medication as a commodity to be maximized for profit. Likewise, the principal question cannot be: "Does this medication work?" if the definition of what "work" means is unclear. Does "work" mean controlling symptoms? Does "work" mean making life easier for the individual? Does "work" mean making life easier for families? Does "work" mean making life easier for society? Or does "work" mean helping the individual renegotiate their relational connectedness with God, others, and themselves in ways that bring about life in all of its fullness—shalom? Such questions draw our attention not only to what medication *does* in a biomedical sense, but also to what it *means* within the life of the individual and those around her. While all these aspects of what "works" may be important, the issue of meaning and the implications of the impact of the drug for someone's personhood are the overarching theological priorities, and this is what should give the other forms of what "works" their intention and goal.

If we are to decommodify our thinking around psychopharmacology and offer a kinder, gentler way of framing medication and the practice of medicating, there are four questions a prescriber might want to bear in mind:

(1) In what sense does this medication facilitate a person's movement back into relationship with God, self, and others?

(2) For whose benefit is this medication prescribed, bought, and administered (the individual, the family, society, the physician, the drug company)?

(3) What will a person gain by the administration/use of this medication?

(4) What will a person lose by the administration/use of this medication?

These kinds of questions enable prescribers to avoid treating patients as mere units and allow patients to benefit from medication in a way that considers the entirety of their lives.

Integrating decommodified thinking in secular systems

The theological framing of psychopharmacology raises an important question: How can its principles be applied in secular systems where explicit consideration of God is absent from the prescribing process? While secular frameworks may not adopt theological language or goals, they can still benefit from decommodified thinking by embracing holistic, person-centered care that prioritizes relational and communal well-being. Secular systems can incorporate these ideas through collaborative models of care. For instance, pairing medication with contributions from chaplaincy, spiritual direction, or other forms of holistic support can foster a more integrated approach to mental health. Chaplains, spiritual directors, and community leaders can work alongside medical professionals to ensure that patients are not only treated for symptoms but are also supported in addressing the relational and existential dimensions of their well-being. These partnerships enable the inclusion of spiritual care and relational healing in treatment plans without imposing any specific theological framework.

Pastors and local churches play an equally significant role in this integrated model. While not medical professionals or institutions, they can create spaces of belonging and spiritual support that complement medical care. Churches can serve as sanctuaries for those navigating mental health challenges, offering community, prayer, and relational care that align with the broader goals of shalom. Pastors can also collaborate with healthcare providers by advocating for patients and ensuring their spiritual and relational needs are acknowledged as part of their overall care.

Additionally, churches can educate their communities about mental health in ways that reduce stigma and promote understanding. By fostering a theology of kindness and relational care, they can help create environments where medication and other treatments are seen not as threats or sources of shame but as tools that enable fuller participation in relationships with God, self, and others.

Decommodification as a vital mental healthcare practice

This kind of decommodified thinking extends beyond prescribing medication; it can also inform counseling, resilience-building, and other mental healthcare practices. To guide these efforts we must ask key questions: Are we using a theological anthropology of kindness to discern both the root causes of people's struggles and the goals of our practices? Or are we, perhaps unintentionally, focusing solely on helping individuals adapt to unjust and oppressive systems? While helping people cope with unjust systems is often necessary and compassionate, it is not sufficient. Those broken by such systems need both healing and hope. Jesus's ministry of healing demonstrates the importance of addressing the immediate needs of individuals caught in unjust social and spiritual frameworks, even as we work toward the broader, long-term goal of transforming those systems. For this reason, mental health ministry should be understood corporately, as part of the church's wider mission to the world—a mission grounded in justice, fairness, and resistance to oppressive structures. Decommodification is not merely about individual practices like counseling, prescribing, or resilience-building; it is about recognizing these practices as interconnected dimensions of the church's commitment to fostering shalom in a fractured world. Decommodifying our minds is itself an act of resistance: it renews our capacity to imagine, to hope, and to act differently within a broken world. Even when systemic change seems beyond our immediate reach, the refusal to internalize the logic of commodification is a vital form of fidelity to the vision of shalom.

HEALING THE SYMPTOM POOL: HELPING PEOPLE LIVE WELL EVEN IN THE MIDST OF SUFFERING AND DISTRESS

In the first chapter I suggested that understanding shalom as mental health makes it possible to find mental health even when others may assume you are mentally unhealthy. Health is marked not by the absence of symptoms, but by the presence of Jesus. Even when symptoms are present, connection with Jesus (mental health) remains a possibility. This leads to an understanding of healing in which the primary objective may not simply be to eradicate symptoms but rather to help people live well with them, with "living well" relating to obtaining and retaining harmony and relationships. Healing, then, is an orientation toward the goal of God's creatures: to live well with God, with one another, and with the various dimensions of creation. This means recognizing the constructive nature of the symptom pool. It means working toward healing destructive constructions and ways of understanding and responding to symptoms that separate people from people and from God.

In chapter 3 I highlighted how mental distress is not just a biological or psychological reality—it is culturally shaped by the language we use to describe it. The concept of the symptom pool suggests that the way we name and interpret suffering profoundly influences how people experience their own mental health challenges. Unkindness, then, is not only about *what we do* but also about *how we speak*. Naming someone's distress in ways that rob them of dignity—reducing their struggle to mere pathology, imposing narrow categories that deny the complexity of their experience—can deepen suffering rather than alleviate it. Conversely, kindness in mental healthcare involves the radical re-humanization of distress. It means naming suffering in ways that allow for agency, hope, and communal belonging. If mental healthcare is to reflect the shalomic vision of wholeness, it must begin by changing the language through which suffering is understood. The example of schizophrenia will help make this point.

Kindness and schizophrenia

As previously argued, aspects of Western culture are pathology-forming. Nowhere is this clearer than in the phenomenon of stigma. Stigma emerges when symptoms associated with mental ill-health are removed from their medico-psychiatric context and weaponized to redefine persons negatively. It is a profoundly unkind act that fractures shalom and wounds personhood. Resistance to such distortion demands reframing the symptom pool: interpreting symptoms in ways that orient towards kindness rather than oppression. Nowhere is this more vital than in the experience of schizophrenia, a condition that powerfully transgresses Western norms about mind, self, and human dignity.

In Western contexts, schizophrenia is intensely stigmatized and feared. Individuals who see and hear realities others do not are framed as "out of their minds," alien to the normal standards of mind and reason. As Ethan Watters notes, even biological explanations cannot wholly sever the cultural assumptions that equate selfhood with internal control and cognitive stability:

> Our biomedical advances are hard to separate from our particular cultural beliefs. It is difficult to distinguish, for example, the biomedical conception of schizophrenia—the idea that the disease exists within the biochemistry of the brain—from the more inchoate Western assumption that the self resides there as well. Mental illness is feared and has such a stigma because it represents a reversal of what Western humans . . . have come to value as the essence of human nature . . . Because our culture so highly values . . . an illusion of self-control and control of circumstance, we become abject when contemplating mentation that seems more changeable, less restrained and less controllable, more open to outside influence, than we imagine our own to be.[11]

[11] Ethan Watters, "The Americanization of Mental Illness," *New York Times Magazine*, January 8, 2010, https://www.nytimes.com/2010/01/10/magazine/10psyche-t.html.

Schizophrenia disrupts the Western illusion of the autonomous, bounded self and in doing so, provokes fear, alienation, and unkindness. Yet this reaction is culturally specific. Tanya Luhrmann's work reveals that in Indian and African cultures, schizophrenia is framed more gently.[12] The expectation of incurable illness is absent; individuals remain within their communities, retaining access to social goods such as work, friendship, and respect. Hearing voices is understood within a more porous theory of mind, where connection to ancestors or the divine is normal, not terrifying. In such contexts, kindness—not fear—becomes the dominant response.

This contrast is theologically significant. It suggests that stigma is not an inevitable feature of mental ill-health, but a contingent, cultural betrayal of kindness. When communities interpret symptoms relationally and generously, outcomes are radically different. As Amy Sousa discovered in her work among families living with people with schizophrenia in India, families and individuals didn't think of themselves as having a career-ending illness. *They expected to recover*. "And, at least in comparison with

[12] Tanya Luhrmann, M. R. Padmavati, Hema Tharoor, and Akwasi Osei, "Hearing Voices in Different Cultures: A Social Kindling Hypothesis," *Topics in Cognitive Science* 7, no. 4 (2015): 646–63, doi:10.1111/tops.12158.

Western people with schizophrenia, they did."[13] The critical point is this: *While symptoms can be intrinsically distressing, cultural interpretation often amplifies suffering and alienation, either deepening the pain or offering pathways toward kindness and hope.*

[13] T. M. Luhrmann and Jocelyn Marrow, *Our Most Troubling Madness: Case Studies in Schizophrenia Across Cultures* (University of California Press, 2017). Although we can't discuss it at great length here, there are some interesting connections here in relation to mental health. It has, for example, been suggested that the kind of social pressure on minority groups caused by a failure to thrive within the kind of economic system we described in the previous chapter can lead to a situation of "social defeat." The theory of social defeat proposes that when a person is placed in a situation where they lose power, status, and self-esteem due to verbal, physical, or psychological abuse, they will essentially give up, overwhelmed with hopelessness, anxiety, and an overpowering sense of helplessness. People who are socially defeated may also show increased aggression towards others. This theory has been suggested as one reason why people of color and immigrants have higher rates of schizophrenia than white Westerners. It may also add to our understanding of violence among young Black African American men in the United States and Afro-Caribbean men in the United Kingdom. If the system defeats you, what do you do? If there is no space for you, where do you find home? See J. P. Selten, E. van der Ven, B. P. Rutten, and E. Cantor-Graae, "The Social Defeat Hypothesis of Schizophrenia: An Update," *Schizophrenia Bulletin* 39, no. 6 (2013): 1180–86, doi:10.1093/schbul/sbt134.

Schizophrenia and the Western mind

At least some of the cultural alienation of schizophrenia rests upon specific Western assumptions about mind and self. As we have discussed, the Western model presumes a closed, bounded, autonomous, and interior mind. Voice-hearing ruptures this model, and so the person is imagined as "not our kind." However, if we refuse this anthropology, if we think with a Christian theory of mind in which the self is already relational, open to God's voice and others, then the alienness of symptoms diminishes. It is true that experiences such as hearing things others do not are unusual. However, (a) the experience of voice-hearing is shared by a significant percentage of the nonpsychiatric population, that is, people who have no diagnosis and are not formally in touch with mental health services;[14] and (b) as we have seen, Christians have similar experiences of hearing voices and a different theory of mind. Viewed in this way, the "symptom"[15] of voice-hearing does not indicate

[14] Catherine Lawrence, Jason Jones, and Myra Cooper, "Hearing Voices in a Non-Psychiatric Population," *Behavioural and Cognitive Psychotherapy* 38, no. 3 (2010): 363–73, https://doi.org/10.1017/S1352465810000172.

[15] I put "symptoms" in quotation marks here as many voice hearers do not frame their experience in terms of symptoms.

that people are "out of their minds." Voice-hearing is unusual, but not incomprehensible. The phenomenon is not as alien or as terrifying as many of us might presuppose. Persons living with schizophrenia are not "outside" humanity. They are our kind. They deserve, and require, kind-ness.

Renaming symptoms

Healing the symptom pool means naming things differently. If we change the way we name the symptom, we change the way it is understood. Using the medical term *hallucinations* indicates an experience is a meaningless symptom. However, if we change the name of the symptom to *voice-hearing*, as I have here, we find ourselves drawn into a more relational frame. People hear voices, and often these voices are meaningful, relational, and significant. Yes, the voices can be disturbing and abusive, but sometimes they are peaceable and supportive.[16] The simple shift in terminology from hallucinations to hearing voices personalizes the "symptom," draws out its relational aspects, and offers a different option for the symptom pool. This in turn offers different ways of

[16] For more on this supportive dimension of voices, see John Swinton, *Finding Jesus in the Storm: The Spiritual Lives of Christians with Mental Health Challenges* (Eerdmans, 2020), ch. 7.

responding. Medication may be necessary, but helping people manage their voices in ways that enable them to live healthily in the midst of difficulties is also an option. The organization called the Hearing Voices Network does precisely this by creating communities of voice hearers who meet together to share their experiences and to learn from one another how to manage their voices.[17]

People living with schizophrenia or any other form of mental health challenges need understanding, kindness, friendship, and a way of revisioning the symptom pool that reminds people of the centrality of kind-ness. *Kindness reinforces kind-ness.* Yes, people have experiences that can be disturbing. That is why the practice and presence of mental health professionals is so vitally important. But such experiences need not prevent people from living well even in the midst of disturbance. Helping people find Jesus in the storm is one of the key gifts the

[17] The Hearing Voices Network (HVN) is a charitable organization based *inter alia* in London, dedicated to supporting individuals who hear voices, see visions, or experience other unusual perceptions. HVN aims to create respectful and empowering spaces, challenge negative stereotypes, and promote a positive understanding of these experiences. They provide information and support and facilitate self-help groups across the United Kingdom and beyond.

church brings to the table of mental healing. Such gift-giving is the very essence of shalom as mental health. Within shalom, people can recover *if* recovery is understood as finding a place of sanctuary, belonging, and hope where they can live well even amidst their wildest storms.

LEARNING TO LOVE OUR FUTURE NEIGHBORS

Finally, the focus on the ecological dimensions of shalom and mental healthcare reminds us not only of the importance of caring for creation but also of the significance of recognizing the eschatological dimensions of mental health and mental healthcare. A temptation when we think about mental healthcare is to focus on the immediate problems, that is, the ways in which we can help the people before us who are struggling with their mental health. This makes sense, and we *absolutely* should do this to the best of our ability. God calls us to offer love and kindness to those we encounter in this moment. Jesus's command to "love your neighbor as yourself" is unchangeable. *People matter now.*

Nonetheless, shalom is an eschatological concept, and so is mental healthcare. Mental health *now* is essential, but mental health in the lives of those who come after us is equally as important. We are called to love our neighbor now, and we are also called to love our future neighbors. That means making sure the world God loved so that he gave us Jesus (John 3:16) is a place fit for the purposes of future life and shalomic love. God calls us to forms of eschatological love which value creation now and which desire to ensure that the gift of creation remains healthy, available, and beautiful for our future neighbors.

This requires that we decommodify our view of the planet, moving away from the commodification of the world toward a perspective on creation as a *gift* that God gives to us and asks us to care for and treat with tenderness and love (Gen 2:15). Rodney Clapp urges us to think beyond the instrumentality of a neoliberal worldview:

> In stark contrast to the anthropocentric preoccupations of both modernity and postmodernity, biblical faith affirms that creation is an eloquent gift of extravagant love. This is not a world of objects that sit mutely waiting for the human subject to master them. Instead, this is a world of created fellow subjects, all called into being by the same Creator, all born of the Creator's love, all included in the Creator's covenant of creational restoration, and all responsive agents in the kingdom of the beloved Son. . . . A creation called into being by the Word of God,

> created in, through and for Christ in whom all creation coheres, is not a mechanistic system but a dynamic, personal, living creation that has a voice.[18]

When creation is perceived as a gift to be received and a mutual duty to be lived out, the idea of commodifying it for the sake of profit inevitably becomes deeply dissonant.

MOVING FORWARD IN KINDNESS

Throughout this book, I have argued that faithful mental healthcare cannot rest upon the fragile scaffolding of individual resilience but must be reimagined through a theological vision of communal healing. If, as I have contended in chapter 2, human minds are relationally constituted and inescapably intertwined, then kindness is not merely a moral duty but a form of participation in the redemptive work of Christ. To practice kindness is to labor for the restoration of shalom; to refuse it is to collude in the fragmentation of minds, bodies, and creation itself. The Christian vision of mental health, shaped by the mind of Christ and oriented toward the eschatological peace of God, calls us not to adjust

[18] Rodney Clapp, *Naming Neoliberalism: Exposing the Spirit of Our Age* (Fortress, 2021), 152.

ourselves to the deformities of a fallen world but to anticipate, even now, the reconciliation of all things. True healing is not found only in helping individuals survive within disordered systems (this side of the eschaton survival remains a task), but also in becoming agents of a new creation, a people among whom peace is made visible within ourselves, between ourselves, with the earth, and with the living God.

POSTSCRIPT

Being Where Our Feet Are

In 2021 I joined a group of musicians called The Porter's Gate[1] for a songwriting project on beautiful Keates Island, just off Vancouver. The meeting was organized by Sanctuary Mental Health Ministries,[2] a Vancouver-based organization focused on enabling churches to care well for people living with mental health challenges. The intention was to write an album of worship songs focused on the lived experience of people with mental health challenges. The album *Sanctuary Songs* was released in 2023 and is, I hope, helping people worship well in difficult

[1] The Porter's Gate Worship Project, https://www.portersgateworship.com/.

[2] Sanctuary Mental Health Ministries, https://sanctuarymentalhealth.org/uk/.

times. One of the songs we wrote is titled "Centering Prayer." The chorus runs like this:

> I wanna be where my feet are.
> I wanna breathe the life around me.
> I wanna listen as my heart beats, right on
>   time.
> I wanna be where my feet are.

It's a lovely and deeply evocative song about the importance of recognizing where we are in this moment, of realizing where our feet are rooted and planted and what that means for the ways in which we encounter God's good creation. I'm very much an urbanite. I tend not to think deeply about my relationship with the land or the importance of the ground on which I stand. I imagine that if I lived in the countryside I would see things differently. Whether we are urbanites or country people, we need to learn to be where our feet are. We need to learn what it means to be truly present in the world and to walk with God through creation.

We have seen the dangers of commodifying the world and the power our destruction of creation has to damage our mental health. If we are to live as shalom people, we need to decommodify our thinking about the world. The first step (literally) toward such a goal is to feel, touch, and learn to love the ground on which we are standing. The ground on which we stand is holy ground, created matter that matters. When we learn to respect the land, accept it as a gift, and realize the importance of being present within and upon it, the possibility of reconnecting with it and acting differently toward it becomes imaginable. Decommodifying the land and noticing where our feet are reminds us of our kinship with the land and helps us treat creation kindly. There is much more to be said on this, but for now, realizing that self-awareness is the first step toward moving from ecological homelessness to spiritual homefulness will at least get us on the road toward actualizing this dimension of shalom.

In this book I have tried to show the importance of looking inward, looking outward, and looking upward for the ways in which we understand and respond to mental health issues and develop mental healthcare strategies. Reflecting on the kindness of Jesus, who is and who brings shalom, provides us a theological framework to begin this vital work of reconnection, harmonizing, and healing. I'll conclude with the words from another of the songs from the Porter's Gate album I mentioned above, which I had the pleasure of cowriting:

> You are my sanctuary,
> my hiding place where I belong.
> You are my peaceful harbor,
> You will bring me safely home.

I think that is true. Life is full of storms. We need a place of sanctuary. We need peace. We need shalom. We need Jesus. He will bring us safely home.

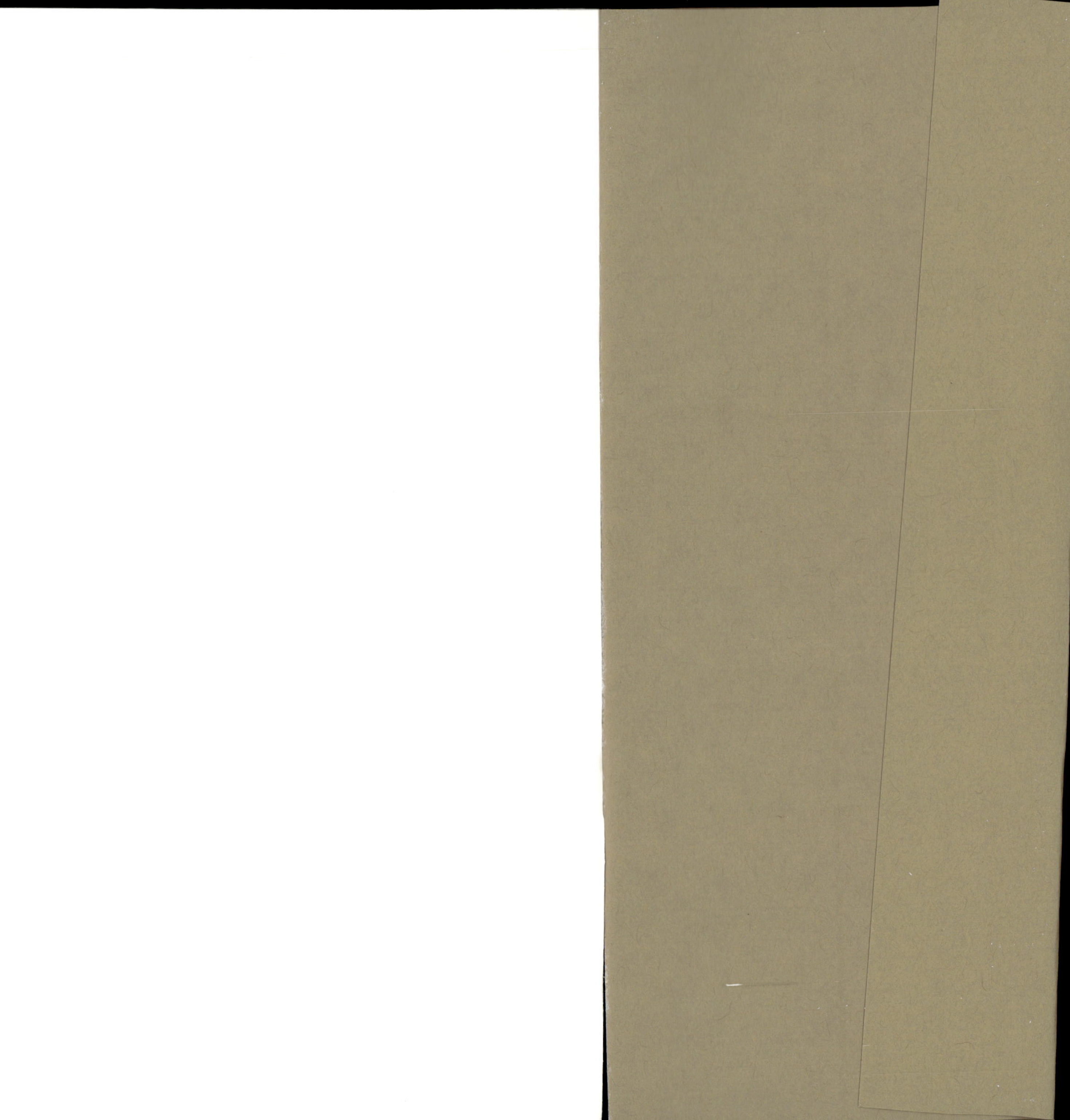